Psychopharmacology

Straight Talk on
Mental Health Medications

Third Edition

Psychosis - Depression - Bipolar
Anxiety - ADHD - Insomnia

Joe Wegmann, RPh, LCSW

Published by
PESI Publishing & Media
PESI, Inc
3839 White Ave
Eau Claire, WI 54703

Cover Design: Amy Rubenzer
Layout Design: Bookmasters & Amy Rubenzer
Edited By: Marietta Whittlesey

Printed in the United States of America

ISBN: 978-1-55957-021-3

Library of Congress Cataloging-in-Publication Data

Wegmann, Joseph.
  Psychopharmacology : straight talk on mental health medications / Joseph Wegmann,
  R.Ph., LCSW. -- Third edition.
     pages cm
  Includes bibliographical references and index.
  ISBN 978-1-55957-021-3 (alk. paper)

1. Psychopharmacology. 2. Mental illness--Chemotherapy. I. Title.
  RM315.W43 2015
  615.7'8--dc23
                                                         2015021937

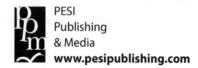

PESI
Publishing
& Media
www.pesipublishing.com

Disclaimer

The material presented in this book is for educational purposes only and should never replace the advice or treatment plan of a physician or other health care practitioner. It should not be used for diagnostic or prescribing purposes. The author offers no endorsement of products, recommendations for drug dosing, or any implied promise of relief. Case studies throughout the book are for illustrative purposes only and are not to be used as models for medication management of a particular disorder. Every attempt was made to present accurate information at the time of publication, but the subject of psychopharmacology is an ever-expanding one. The author assumes no responsibility or liability for any action taken as a result of the information contained in this book.

Acknowledgment

B,
Thanks for the willingness to do, as you put it, "whatever it takes" to help make this book a success. I am most grateful.
UNC

The Author

Who Is He, and What Does He Do?

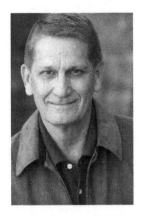

Joe Wegmann is a licensed clinical pharmacist and clinical social worker with more than thirty years of experience in the field of psychopharmacology. His diverse professional background in psychopharmacology and psychotherapy affords him a unique perspective on medication management issues. Joe is well known for the practical, relevant and insightful psychopharmacology seminars he conducts across the country. Joe has written eight books on psychiatric medication management—including the best seller *Psychopharmacology Straight Talk on Mental Health Medications*, now in its third edition. He writes columns, articles and blogs for his website *www.pharmatherapist.com*, *Psychology Today*, *Social Work Today*, *Woman's World* and many others. Joe served as Adjunct Professor of Psychopharmacology in the Master of Social Work program at Southern University of New Orleans for 17 years and maintains an active psychotherapy practice specializing in the treatment of depression and anxiety

Table of Contents

SECTION FOUR
Specific Populations, ADHD, Herbals & Supplements, Solving Medication Challenges

APPENDICES

The Bigger Picture and What's Inside

With medication management playing an increasingly pivotal role in the treatment of mental health disorders, the challenges faced by clinicians are increasing. For one, non-medical clinicians provide the majority of mental health services in the United States. For another, the majority of prescriptions and orders for psychotropic medications are written <u>not</u> by psychiatrists, but by family practice and primary care physicians. As a result, you may be working with patients who are neither in a program of monitored drug use nor being treated with a combination of medication and psychotherapy.

Under these conditions, it is essential for all healthcare professionals, particularly those providing mental health services, to have a working knowledge of psychotropic medications. Ideally, medication prescribers and non-prescribers alike will work together to implement treatment strategies and improve clinical outcomes.

This book follows a straightforward, user-friendly format. It first provides a summary of disorders you might routinely encounter -including psychoses, depression, bipolar and anxiety; followed by a discussion of the medication management of these disorders. This book also examines pharmacotherapy in special population groups, specifically, children and adolescents, pregnant women and geriatric patients.

Select topics are also discussed—including treatment-resistant depression, issues linked to noncompliance, and what you as a practitioner can do to address noncompliance.

With many people self-medicating with herbal remedies, dietary supplements and vitamins, this book also outlines the herbal treatments that have proven beneficial in treatment and those that pose potentially harmful interactions with prescription drugs.

Here's hoping that this unique and practical book will assist you in gaining a comprehensive understanding of the mechanisms of action, clinical applications, common adverse effects and risks of the medications most frequently prescribed in the contemporary treatment of psychiatric disorders. The goal of this book is to guide you in practical and clinically relevant language through the maze of mental health medications, then help you identify ways to use your expanded knowledge to improve client outcomes. (Throughout the text, the terms "patient" and "client" will be used interchangeably depending on the context of the discussion, but essentially mean the same thing.)

New to the Third Edition

Thank you for choosing this fully revised and updated third edition of *Psychopharmacology: Straight Talk On Mental Health Medications*. Building on the strengths of its second edition predecessor, this edition broadens its scope by including the most current updates on the assessment and diagnosis of the mental health syndromes most frequently encountered in clinical practice— psychosis, depression, bipolar, anxiety and ADHD. Recent advances in the medication management of these disorders are discussed at length and all new psychiatric medication releases are included. Key to the third edition will be in-depth discussions of when and under what circumstances non-pharmacological interventions are the preferred treatment modalities, together with recommendations for how to best utilize medication and psychotherapies in a complementary way.

Also New:

- The nuts and bolts of diagnosis and developing client rapport
- DSM-5 and psychotropic medication prescribing
- Neuroscience—why it's fascinating to read but impractical in the treatment room
- A more detailed look at depression and what perpetuates it
- An expanded section on the risk factors of antidepressants
- Why bipolar disorder treatment remains stuck in neutral
- Anxiety treatment: what should *not* be medicated
- Much expanded section on insomnia
- Updates on herbal and other alternative treatments
- More on additive and combination medication protocols

- Why there's little news on the child and adolescent front
- Geriatric psychopharmacology—the latest and
- Psychotropic medication discontinuation—safe strategies that work.

Psychopharmacology: Straight Talk on Mental Health Medications, Third Edition, is a desk reference suitable for healthcare professionals and for anyone interested in expanding their knowledge of how to best manage mental health maladies both pharmacologically and behaviorally.

Joe Wegmann
New Orleans, LA

SECTION ONE

GETTING STARTED WITH THE CLIENT

CHAPTER 1

The DSM; Medical Model; Neurobiology

Biological psychiatry is a branch of psychiatry that focuses on understanding mental disorders from a biological standpoint. More specifically, it focuses on the functions of the human nervous system. The practice of biological psychiatry—also known as biopsychiatry—dates back to ancient times, yet the term itself was not used until the mid-20th century. That's when the research, creation and use of newly developed drugs intensified, resulting in new classes of pharmacological agents, which addressed mental-health disorders, including tranquilizers, antidepressants and anti-psychotics.

THE DSM

Around the same time that these new drugs were emerging, the need for a dependable body of knowledge that would assist clinicians in defining the approximately 100 diagnostic mental health categories used at the time became clear. In 1952, the first *Diagnostic and Statistical Manual of Mental Health Disorders* was published. Better known by its initials "DSM," the guide is now in its fifth edition—DSM-5.

With the arrival of the DSM, the emphasis shifted away from the psychoanalytically based models and treatments of Freud, Adler and Jung—theorists and clinicians who were more interested in the <u>why</u> of a disorder than its <u>what</u>—to more descriptive and biological models and treatments. Also, where the older psychoanalytic models tended to classify <u>individuals,</u> the DSM classifies <u>disorders.</u> We use the DSM to compare the signs and symptoms of our client presentations through a set of objective criteria. The DSM serves as a guide to clinical practice by helping clinicians define disorders more consistently. This, in turn, allows for a better prediction of prognosis and treatment response.

The DSM-5 was in development for more than 10 years. Its official release was announced in May, 2013 at the American Psychiatric Association's annual meeting in San Francisco, California. New diagnoses have been added and others have been amended or combined. Some proposed criteria considered for inclusion stirred up so much public and professional ire they were eventually eliminated from the final draft.

The most noteworthy changes to the manual are concept-driven. The multiaxial system of the previous DSMs has been dropped in favor of a dimensional diagnostic scheme. This new format combines the former axes I, II, and III with separate notations for psychosocial and context factors (formerly axis IV) and disability (formerly axis V). Also, the Chapter order is different and other disorders have been grouped.

The furor surrounding the DSM-5's changes—particularly its additions—has subsided, for the most part, as of this writing. However, in the first six months subsequent to its release, proponents and opponents of the guide's changes eagerly held their ground, defending their positions. I have conducted my own thorough independent review of the DSM-5, so here's my take on its positives and negatives:

Positives

- The DSM-5 has tightened up criteria in the best interest of patients.
- The multiaxial classification system needed to go. Most of us practice professionals used axes I and II all but exclusively.
- Mental retardation is no longer being used as a diagnosis and is being replaced by "Intellectual Disability." This change comports well with established practices in the field.
- Autistic disorder is gone as a diagnosis and is replaced by "autistic spectrum disorder." Also gone is Asperger Syndrome. This is a good move, because the spectrum concept provides overall better usefulness for the autistic disorders as a group.
- Another positive change is the reorganization of disorders such as Obsessive-Compulsive disorder and Posttraumatic Stress disorder. Anxiety is not the root cause of either of these disorders therefore these syndromes have been re-grouped accordingly as a reflection of clinical advancements aided by neuroscience.
- In the schizophrenia arena, the five subtypes (disorganized, catatonic, undifferentiated, etc.) were nixed because they were largely ignored.

Negatives

- **Disruptive Mood Dysregulation Disorder (DMDD).** This diagnosis morphed out of the over-diagnosis of bipolar disorder in youth, and will serve as a diagnostic dumping ground for children by pathologizing what amounts in many instances to no more than garden variety temper tantrums. We already have Oppositional Defiant disorder to cover for this, and it's quite adequate. And what's the chance that a clinician who is intolerant of unruly behavior will be quick to diagnosis this and get paid by an insurance company? This is a mess waiting to happen, is untested and opens another door for medicating kids inappropriately and excessively.

- **Generalized Anxiety Disorder.** This disorder has had shady boundaries since it was first included in the DSM. Now that the duration of symptoms has been reduced from six months to three months it will be harder to distinguish what is truly a chronic disorder from the concerns of everyday life. This will create a sizable new subset of "anxious" people who may be unnecessarily treated with anti-anxiety medications when all they are experiencing are the ups and downs of living life on life's terms.

- **Bereavement Exclusion.** Widespread criticism emanated from the decision to eliminate the so-called bereavement exclusion in which a grieving individual had up to two months after the death of a loved one without being diagnosed with Major Depressive Disorder. This simply did not need to be meddled with. Grief is an absolutely normal human response to loss and should not be placed on the "clock" so to speak, and any competent clinician wouldn't miss the presence of major depression—even when occurring during bereavement.

- **Attention Deficit Hyperactivity Disorder (ADHD).** The DSM-5 has rendered the path to diagnosing ADHD easier than it has ever been. According to the Centers for Disease Control and Prevention (CDC), nearly one in five high school age boys in the United States and 11 percent of school-age children have received a diagnosis of ADHD. There has been a 53 percent rise in diagnosis in those ages 4–17 in this past decade alone. The DSM-5 allows for symptoms to merely "impact" daily activities, rather than cause impairment. Also, the requirement that symptoms appear before age 7 is changed to before age 12. My number one concern here is that since every psychiatric syndrome on earth adversely affects attention in some way, making it easier to go to ADHD means that other potentially important diagnoses may be overlooked.

The DSM has served as a viable diagnostic guide for decades now, and its use as a teaching tool for graduate students and novice clinicians for understanding the process steps pursuant to diagnosis has proven to be most valuable. My overall assessment though is that the diagnostic bar has been lowered, and people with bonafide psychiatric illnesses are already badly shortchanged from a treatment perspective due to our severely fractured mental health system. The DSM-5 will make this worse by directing scarce resources away from the very ill and instead toward people mislabeled as mentally ill.

MEDICAL MODEL

Since the age of Hippocrates, medication has been used to manage both physical and mental-health pathologies. The primary goal of the medical model is to identify these pathologies and then attempt to fix them. This is as true today as it was 2,500 years ago. Over time, three goals of pharmacotherapy have emerged: 1) to treat an acute disorder; 2) to prevent relapse after clinical improvement; and 3) to prevent future episodes of the disorder. More simply described, these are the acute, continuation and maintenance goals of medication management:

> **Acute treatment** is initiated to ameliorate the symptoms of an actively occurring disorder. During this phase, the primary goal is to stabilize the patient using medication. Acute treatment begins with the initial prescribing of medication, and generally lasts for a period of up to six months of prescribed use, according to the National Institute of Mental Health (NIMH).

> **Continuation treatment** is utilized to prevent relapse after the initial improvement. Here, the goal is to minimize the possibility of patient decompensation after stabilization. This period of medication use extends from six months to one year, as defined by the NIMH.

> **Maintenance treatment** is utilized to prevent future episodes of a disorder. Two acceptable examples of this pharmacotherapy goal are the use of mood stabilizers for bipolar disorder and antipsychotics for schizophrenia. While the NIMH defines this phase as prescribed drug use for a period of one to two years, several disorders discussed in this book are linked to long-term and even lifetime prevalence of psychotropic medication utilization.

BIOLOGY OF PSYCHOPHARMACOLOGY

Pharmacokinetics

Pharmacokinetics, or the study of what the body does to a drug, is associated with four basic processes: absorption, distribution, metabolism and excretion.

Absorption is the movement of a substance into the bloodstream. In other words, this is the process of a substance entering the body.

Distribution involves the scattering of drugs or substances throughout body tissues and fluids.

Metabolism is the transformation or breakdown of substances such that they are prepared for elimination from the body. Metabolism occurs primarily in the liver.

Excretion is the process by which substances leave the body. Excretion occurs primarily through the kidneys.

Pharmacodynamics

Pharmacodynamics is the science of drug action. Basically, it studies what a drug does to the body. More specifically, pharmacodynamics studies the mechanism of a drug action and the relationship between drug concentration and effect.

The effects that any drug has on the body may be intended or unintended. In a "perfect drug" scenario, medications would zero in on only their intended target systems, generate only desired effects, then metabolize and leave the body. But as almost everyone who has ever taken medications knows, drugs have unintended and undesirable effects as well. In this sense, they take a shotgun approach rather than a rifle approach to the body in that hopefully we get what we want from them, but at the same time unfortunately get some of what we don't want as well. For all of us, the most desired effect of any medication is its pharmacological effect, namely, does the drug actually <u>do</u> what it claims to do. Undesirable consequences of medication use include side effects, allergic reactions, rare yet potentially serious unpredictable events such as anaphylaxis, and the effects on the body if a drug is abruptly discontinued.

Later on in this book, recommendations for the dosing and scheduling of medications in special population groups such as expectant mothers, children, adolescents and older adults will also be discussed. Yet another challenge facing prescribers in the future will be how to appropriately address the way that different ethnic groups respond to medication. There is evidence suggesting that several psychotropic medication classes are metabolized differently, thereby producing different response rates when prescribed to African Americans and Asians, for example. This suggests that accepted dosing practices may require modification when prescribed to those in different ethnic groups.

DRUG INTERACTIONS

A detailed discussion of the various types of pharmacokinetic and pharmacodynamic interactions is beyond the intent of this book, but it's beneficial to have a working knowledge of what happens when drugs enter the system and what their effects are on other drugs and even foodstuffs that are also consumed. Pharmacokinetic interactions involve the absorption, distribution, metabolism and excretion processes described above, or more specifically, what the body does to a drug.

Drug-food interactions are more prevalent than drug-drug interactions during the absorption process. For example, the absorption of the antipsychotic drug Geodon (ziprasidone), discussed in Chapter 7, is slowed if taken without food. Thus, Geodon (ziprasidone) users are advised to take the drug after a meal.

An example of a distribution process interaction would be taking Depakote (divalproex), discussed in Chapter 11, and aspirin together. In this instance, aspirin displaces a portion of the Depakote (divalproex) from its protein binding, causing the unbound Depakote (divalproex) portion to increase, resulting in increased Depakote (divalproex) levels.

During the metabolism process, drugs are broken down by enzymes in a number of different ways to facilitate their elimination from the body via either the urine or feces.

An excretion process example would be the use of lithium together with caffeinated beverages or energy drinks. Caffeinated coffee or tea accelerate kidney function and can lead to decreased lithium levels.

Pharmacodynamic interactions involve the effect(s) that drugs have on the body when taken together. An example would be the use of a benzodiazepine drug such as Valium (diazepam) taken together with an antihistamine drug such as Benadryl (diphenhydramine). Each of these taken separately can cause drowsiness, but when taken concomitantly, the user can become markedly drowsy. Both drugs are discussed in Chapter 12.

Interactions happen because of misinformation, misuse or often in instances where little or no guidance is provided at all. Interactions among drugs, foods or medicinal plants and herbs run the gamut from benign to potentially fatal. Fortunately very few are lethal, and many drug-drug interactions can be managed via dosage titration upward or downward. The major risk factors are toxicity when drug actions are synergistic and a lack of therapeutic efficacy when actions are antagonistic. And of course, there's the ever-present risk of worsening side effects when drugs are combined.

Psychotropic Medication Drug Interactions Worth Noting

- Antidepressants, antipsychotics and some of the older anticonvulsants are linked to significant drug interactions, so be on alert if your patient is taking any of these drug classes.

- Be on alert for the drugs with narrow therapeutic indexes, namely when the toxic dose and the therapeutic dose are in close proximity to one another. Examples include: Lithium, Tegretol (carbamazepine), as well as medications often used in physical medicine such as the blood thinner Warfarin, the cardio active drug Digoxin and the anticonvulsant Dilantin (phenytoin).

- Be aware that the risk of drug interactions increases as the number of medications the patient is taking increases. This can be of significant importance in elderly and pediatric populations.

NEUROTRANSMITTERS

Neurotransmitters are chemicals associated with a complex series of nerve pathways that regulate what we humans think, feel and do. Medical experts have identified as many as 50 peptide neurotransmitters that have been shown to exert their effects on nerve cell function. There are probably many more as yet undiscovered, since the brain contains approximately 100 billion neurons, or nerve cells, that are regulated by these neurotransmitters. The six neurotransmitters that are most important to psychopharmacology are: norepinephrine, serotonin, dopamine, gamma-aminobutyric acid (GABA), acetylcholine and glutamate.

> **Norepinephrine (noradrenalin)** is a hormone secreted by the adrenal glands in response to stress or arousal. It is the principal neurotransmitter of sympathetic nerve endings supplying the major organs and skin. Norepinephrine regulates alertness, anxiety, tension, and the ability to have positive feelings. It is also linked to the mobilization of the body's resources during the activation of the "fight or flight" response. As such, it is released in response to an imminent danger or threat, resulting in an increase in heart rate, blood pressure and respiration. Elevated levels of norepinephrine can lead to states of increased anxiety and, in some cases, mania. Low levels of norepinephrine are implicated in depression.

> **Serotonin** is a vasoconstrictor present in blood serum that is linked to the regulation of mood, anger, aggression, anxiety, appetite, learning, sleep, sexual functioning, states of consciousness and pain. Low

levels of brain serotonin are associated with clinical depression, obsessive compulsive disorder and anxiety disorders. Selective serotonin reuptake inhibitors (SSRIs), a class of antidepressants specific to serotonin regulation, will be discussed in Chapter 5.

Dopamine influences emotional behavior and cognition, and it regulates motor and endocrine activity, among other factors. It has numerous important roles in brain function, including attention, mood, sociability, motivation, desire, pleasure and learning. Dopamine is also strongly associated with reward mechanisms in the brain. Unusually high dopamine action can lead to psychoses and schizophrenia; many antipsychotic medications are formulated to block excess dopamine

Gamma-aminobutyric acid (GABA) is an amino acid that is the central nervous system's major inhibitory neurotransmitter. GABA regulation is associated with emotional balance, sleep patterns and anxiety. Low GABA levels in the limbic system—the "emotional brain"—are associated with increased anxiety, irritability and agitation. GABA activation results in decreased anxiety. This process can be facilitated through the use of benzodiazepine anti-anxiety agents, including Ativan (lorazepam), Xanax (alprazolam) and Valium (diazepam), as well as through the use of mood-stabilizing neuromodulators such as Tegretol (carbamazepine) and Depakote (divalproex). All of these drugs act to calm overall brain excitation.

Acetylcholine was the first neurotransmitter to be identified; it was discovered in the early 1900s. This neurotransmitter is released through the stimulation of the vagus nerve, which alters heart-muscle contractility. Acetylcholine is also important to functional memory, and it has been the subject of much of the research investigating cognitive dysfunction and memory deficits linked to Alzheimer's disease and other organic brain syndromes. The inhibitory or "blocking" actions of certain antidepressants on acetylcholine will be addressed in Chapter 5.

Glutamate is the brain's primary excitatory neurotransmitter. It is a basic building block of proteins and plays an important role in learning and memory.

A FEW WORDS ABOUT NEUROSCIENCE AND EVIDENCE-BASED MEDICINE

The brain is far more complex than the body and it will take decades to ascertain what its capabilities are. So as fascinating as neuroscience and a gaze into the future can be to read about, it's impractical in the treatment room because we treat in the here and now. Neuroscientific development moves at a "laboratory" pace—which is very slow—and is high on the list to fall prey to the vagaries of funding. It has been known to disappoint often as the mysteries of brain functioning have defeated the DSMs and even the best NIMH efforts in search of valid and reliable biomarkers. Progress toward a clearer understanding of mental disorders will be painstaking. To use baseball references: there will be no grand slam home runs; there will be some singles, maybe the occasional double and triple and lots of strikeouts. This phenomenon is true of all of medicine however. We're obviously still fighting the war on cancer and losing most of the battles, so it will be several orders of difficulty more challenging to figure out schizophrenia.

RESEARCH STUDIES

Beware of the words "studies show" or "clinical evidence indicates." Evidence-based medicine is valuable only to the degree that what is presented is done so in a thorough, encompassing way. Many of the studies about what is trending in the Psychopharmacology field aren't worth the paper they are written on or the cyberspace in which they have been transmitted. Take the FDA approval process for example. All that is needed to pass FDA muster is that a potential new drug candidate outperform placebo. The fact is many of these drugs are weakly beating placebo! We're supposed to be excited about that? What's most important is how well a possible newcomer stacks up against the existing competition. That is, you want to know how it ranks head-to-head compared to other established agents within the genre. This is a real weakness with the FDA approval process, and it's an issue with all medication classes within the bounds of physical and mental health medicine.

As consumers, when we're bombarded by direct-to-consumer advertising to buy something, we often become wary because we have learned the importance of protecting ourselves against misrepresentation and sham products. By contrast, we healthcare professionals tend to have very little skepticism when it comes to what we read and digest in medical and scientific journals. Realize that the peer review system is not perfect and is subject to publication bias and that a study which reads professionally and is footnoted to the hilt doesn't necessarily render it credible. "Studies" and "clinical evidence" should be but one component of your overall decision-making. Also, look for who published the data—that is, consider the source. If the authors are employees of a pharmaceutical company, or if they are in the company's speakers' stable, be cautious and take those conflicts into account.

CHAPTER 2

The First Visits with the Client

THE NUTS AND BOLTS OF ASSESSMENT AND DIAGNOSIS

The skilled mental health diagnostician is not seeking perfection as there is no such thing. Instead, this clinician is seeking diagnostic assuredness. Success is the goal. And success is defined in terms of whether the client's position (or condition, if you'd rather) has improved as a result of the professional encounter. Nothing else really matters.

Diagnosing mental health conditions is more art than science—always was, always will be. The diagnosis of general medical conditions is not without an art component, but physical medicine has a major advantage over mental health medicine: the ability to objectify findings. There is an obvious, self-evident advantage to be able to confirm findings by way of blood work, scans and pictures (as in X-rays). In mental health, there is not one single blood test or reliable scan to aid in diagnostic confirmation. It's just the way it is for now, and I suspect for a long time to come.

The diagnostic journey begins with a thorough assessment of the presenting client's situation. The DSM stays on the sidelines, serving only as confirmation and as a reference for coding purposes. Savvy practitioners rely on the "art of the question." That is not to say they don't bring an excellent command of the signs and symptoms of the mental disorder spectrum to the process. They do. But the essence of their skill lies in the ability to frame a series of insightful, intuitive questions around the client's presenting problem. Adroitly, assertively, and yet tactfully, they approach assessment with tactical precision and are aware that success with any client means this: the language controls the discussion; the discussion controls the relationship; and the relationship controls the quality of the outcomes. As such, the highest premium is placed on rapport building. Observation is also important. The nuances of client head movements, facial expressions and overall body language are every bit as important as the changes in their vocal delivery. What these clinicians see in a client is every bit as important to them as what they hear.

Diagnosis then isn't all that complicated when the clinician is asking the right questions, observing appropriately and listening intently. Systematically, the clinician shapes the client's responses and non-verbal behavior—gathered though questioning and aided by insight and intuition—into a diagnosis. The clinician also seeks out collateral sources of information which are supportive of the client's efforts to get better. There is no better way to confirm findings, so they explain to the client that a signed consent permitting outside input is in the best interest of their work together. Then, if the client refuses, that's considered a red flag. Collateral sources are important to the assessment and diagnostic process because lying, minimizing, rationalizing, denying and omission are common to some clients to varying extents. All of the above is pursuant to advancing to the next step—developing a customized, individualized treatment plan with established behavioral objectives that can be measured in terms of progress. It's important to be prescriptive and not solely diagnostic by telling clients what will help them; don't strive to merely achieve consensus with the client. Be the thought leader in the room.

Pros are expected to guide clients toward unburdening themselves as part of assessment, diagnostic and treatment protocols; the heavier lifting though—the change process—is the client's domain. There are numerous variables that impinge upon client symptoms, the most important of which is whether the client is ready to get better. The most renowned clinician on the planet won't make a difference in the uncommitted individual; whereas the clinician with a poor skillset will likely be able to help a highly motivated person at least somewhat.

The skilled clinician approaches each session with a confident presence, secure in his or her abilities and fully present in what is unfolding during the therapeutic encounter. This is the treatment professional who prepares fully, gets up in the morning, shows up, does the best possible, goes home and comes back the next day with the same positive mindset and work ethic.

WHAT IS UNIQUE ABOUT YOUR CLIENT?

When clients first enter your office and you begin building a therapeutic alliance, how do you VIEW them? Are they mostly representative of the signs, symptoms and complaints they present with or do you take into account what they really want from working with you and how their uniqueness—that is "what makes them-them" will determine your approach to working together?

Traditional, evidenced-based treatment interventions follow a consolidation principle. Clients are perceived in terms of their presenting problem and associated symptoms which can range from mild to severe and impact the client as merely annoying or very debilitating; or if medication is deemed necessary, clients are viewed as neurotransmitter-imbalanced or biochemically deficient. Such reductionist approaches focus on ameliorating symptoms that clients often aren't willing to give up and also views them in terms of their similarities, not their differences. We clinicians should ask our clients what they want from treatment and <u>what they may find themselves without</u> if treatment works. For example, a client who professes that he wants to become more independent and self-reliant through treatment and starts to do so, may begin to fear the loss of the support system upon which he has relied heavily in the past, as the system notices his ability to function without its repeated involvement. So, it's important to determine what sets clients apart from one another, recognize this unique specialness and learn about the people most important to them.

DEVELOPING CLIENT RAPPORT

Improving your client's presenting condition—again, the <u>only</u> thing that counts—will not result from how much you know or may think you know, how many workshops you've attended, how many letters you string behind your name or how many certifications you've earned. What matters most is your ability and capacity to develop rapport. And the only way to do this is to be fully present when in the company of the client and to listen closely. The goal is to draw the client in, get them attracted to your maturity, professionalism, enthusiasm and the ease of doing "business" with you. It's not about having all the answers, it's about asking the questions that aid you in assembling the puzzle pieces of the client's situation that are so often vexing. If you ask lousy questions, no matter the response, they won't be useful for reaching the contractual goals you have established with the client system. In most instances, getting to the point of your work together for that day—whether during the first or the twentieth session - is best accomplished by taking a few minutes to chat about something both you and the client enjoy or have in common. This eases the transition to the more serious work yet to come. Also, match your communication style as best you can to the client's. Mimic their speaking rhythm, mannerisms and determine how they learn best. Are they more auditory, visual or kinesthetic?

A touchier issue, difficult for many, is keeping one's mouth shut. You must let the client speak without interruption. Enthusiasm is a core asset, but if unbridled, it can lead to you talking more than the client—a veritable recipe for a poor outcome because you won't learn anything by talking. Other ways and techniques for developing rapport include:

- Dressing professionally
- Displaying symbols of comfort in your office
- Discreetly taking notes during sessions
- Leaning slightly forward when addressing the client as a gesture of interest and
- Continually soliciting the client's beliefs and input when selecting treatment interventions.

Skillfully engaging a client and getting them out of the doom-and-gloom loop and into the success loop is not contingent upon telling them everything you know. It's about telling them what they need to know, pulling them in and getting them to trust that you are the go-to professional for improving their plight.

There are innumerable methodologies, technologies and treatment plans through which effective treatment can be delivered. The key is to have the client perceive these as user-friendly and specific to their situation, not convoluted and complicated. Sounding smart and intelligent is most certainly a plus when delivering services but doesn't necessarily translate into value for the client. Focusing primarily on having a conversation with the client in each session makes it easier for the client to relate to you and be relaxed in your presence. This will place you in a better position to focus on objectives and outcomes by serving as the client's navigational system—their GPS, so to speak. Then with a collective eye on what you and the client have established, help them determine the shortest route possible to getting there.

The most powerful impact you will have on your clients' recovery lies in your ability to foster and sustain hope to heal the wounds of mental illness. Devote attention to focusing and nurturing client strengths and building resilience, and never ever view the client as damaged. People come to treatment for all sorts of reasons. Some are simply stuck and need a nudge; others may be looking for validation and a sounding board; still others are acutely ill. Deliver value to them accordingly and be vigilant about providing outstanding "customer" service by bringing honest, believable energy and enthusiasm to your work. Some clients will need cheerleading and a bit of salesmanship to get them moving, so don't be passive when discussing strategies which you believe can help them—just don't cross the line into coercion. And regardless of how you attempt to help people, compliance with what you are offering is paramount. If the client becomes resistant, find out why as best you can and get them back on track. Lastly, if you dwell on all the clients you don't help, don't try to help themselves, or just drop out of treatment suddenly, you will do a lot of dwelling over a career. These are burnout traps that can derail your career to the extent that you may not be able to recover, so place personal and professional self-care at the head of your priority list to best ensure that as many people as possible can continue to benefit from your expertise.

SECTION TWO

CLINICAL SYNDROMES

CHAPTER 3

Schizophrenia and Other Psychotic Spectrum Disorders

In *Surviving Schizophrenia*, E. Fuller Torrey, M.D., recounts a conversation in which he told a woman that her daughter had schizophrenia. "Anything but that!" the woman replied in horror. "Why couldn't she have leukemia or some other disease?" Dr. Torrey reassured the mother that schizophrenia was much more treatable than a cancer that might cost the girl her life. Yet the woman answered sadly, "I would still prefer that my daughter had leukemia."

Such is the stigma that this psychiatric disorder carries, made worse by the way our society treats those afflicted with it. According to the NIMH, approximately 2.4 million American adults, or about 1.1 percent of the population age 18 and older in a given year, have schizophrenia. An alarming number of homeless people suffer from schizophrenia—perhaps as high as 40 percent, say some statistics—and are likely to be rotated among the streets, shelters, emergency rooms, public psychiatric assistance programs and even the jails. To be sure, those suffering from schizophrenia can have disturbing symptoms. They may hear voices, experience hallucinations, speak incoherently, break out in senseless laughter, and weep and rage without provocation. Prior to 1954 - when Thorazine (chlorpromazine) was approved in the United States for psychiatric treatment - these individuals were certainly feared. Because society couldn't make sense of such behavior, these folks were routinely confined to asylums. Little was known about effective treatment or rehabilitation.

Today, because more has been learned about the brain, nutrition, genetics, environmental factors and of course, new medications and other therapies, the outlook for treating schizophrenia has improved markedly. For diagnostic purposes, clinicians still often use certain criteria to determine which types of psychotic disorders are being presented. More specifically, when the only pathology is the psychotic disorder itself, it is known as a primary psychosis. When the symptoms are a result of a general medical condition or are substance-induced, it is referred to as a secondary psychosis. Also, a distinction is made between psychosis and schizophrenia. Psychosis is a general term that describes psychotic features whereas schizophrenia is a type of psychosis.

MAJOR PSYCHOTIC SPECTRUM DISORDERS

Brief psychotic disorder

This is a psychosis that has a rapid onset and generally follows an identifiable stressor. It is characterized by emotional turmoil, mood changes and confusion, along with the presence of one or more of the following symptoms: delusions, hallucinations, disorganized speech or grossly disorganized or catatonic behavior. Brief psychotic disorder is time-limited, lasting at least one day but less than one month.

Delusional disorder

This involves the presence of sometimes elaborate, non-bizarre delusions—something that could be true, but likely is not after investigation. For example, someone believes that their spouse is having an affair, when in fact the accused has provided ample evidence of their faithfulness. The delusion consumes the lives of these individuals as they become utterly convinced that what they believe is actually happening, despite evidence to the contrary. Delusions are considered bizarre if they are clearly beyond plausibility and not derived from ordinary life events or experiences as in the "affair" example above.

Schizoaffective disorder

With this condition, someone exhibits features of both schizophrenia—delusions, hallucinations and thought distortion—and a mood component, such as depression or mania. The diagnosis is made when the person has features of both illnesses, but does not strictly meet criteria for either schizophrenia or a mood disorder alone. For this reason, achieving diagnostic accuracy is quite difficult. Schizoaffective disorder appears to be about one-third as common as schizophrenia.

Schizophreniform disorder

This is often referred to as a "short episode of schizophrenia." Symptoms are similar to those of schizophrenia; they last at least one month, but less than six months. Roughly half of all those diagnosed with schizpheniform disorder are subsequently diagnosed with schizophrenia.

Schizophrenia

The "granddaddy" of the psychotic spectrum disorders, schizophrenia involves a psychotic phase characterized by prominent psychotic features, such as delusions, hallucinations and gross impairment in reality testing. Continuous signs of these features must persist for at least six months. Schizophrenia also causes social, occupational and other vocational functional impairment that must last for at least six months.

Evidence suggests that schizophrenia has a significant genetic component. Its onset is influenced by psychosocial and environmental factors and stressors. This cruel and chronically debilitating disorder is also a leading cause of disability.

For men, the adult onset age is typically 18 to 20, while for women, it is the mid-twenties. Adolescent age onset typically occurs between the ages of 11–15 for both boys and girls. Childhood-onset schizophrenia is considered rare, with a rate of probability less than 1 in 10,000. Because it is so rare, a detailed history is essential to confirm diagnostic accuracy.

Etiology. From a neurophysiological perspective, several neurotransmitters — most notably dopamine and glutamate—have been implicated in the development of schizophrenia. The hyperactivity of dopamine in the limbic system pathway is a consistent finding. The hypofunction of glutamate could also be responsible for certain aspects of schizophrenia.

Diagnosis. Diagnosing schizophrenia is difficult for several reasons: The disorder is complex, symptoms may appear only briefly, and symptoms may be present in conjunction with other disorders.

Symptoms of Schizophrenia

Positive Symptoms:
- Delusions
- Hallucinations
- Exaggerations in language and communication
- Disorganized speech
- Disorganized behavior

Negative Symptoms:
- Anhedonia (loss of pleasure)
- Emotional withdrawal
- Passivity
- Apathy
- Dulled affect, or "emotional flattening"

Cognitive Symptoms:
- Incoherence
- Loose associations
- Impaired attention
- Impaired information processing

Symptom Domains of Schizophrenia

Positive symptoms are not positive in the ordinary sense of the word. They are described as such because they are the active, observable and treatable symptoms of the disorder. These include both delusions—false fixed beliefs held with conviction—and hallucinations, including auditory, visual and other false and abnormal perceptions.

Negative symptoms aren't considered something "bad." These symptoms refer to things that are "lost" from an affected individual's personality or how life is experienced. These include:

- Blunted affect, which can manifest as a type of "masked," expressionless look
- Emotional withdrawal
- Passivity and apathy and
- Anhedonia, or the inability to experience pleasure

Cognitive Symptoms. Examples of neurocognitive deficits include:
- Impaired executive function: poor problem-solving, reduced capacity to accommodate and assimilate new information
- Attention deficits
- Impaired memory function and
- Impaired informational processing

Those with schizophrenia can become combative, sometimes in conjunction with fear, as a result of hallucinations and delusional or confusing thoughts. This aggression can manifest itself in both verbal and physical attacks, acting out sexually, self-mutilation and suicide attempts. About half of these individuals attempt suicide as a result of "command" delusions, hallucinations or major depression, and 10 percent of them eventually succeed.

Medical Disorders Influencing Psychotic Features
Medical disorders that can influence psychotic manifestations must be ruled out in order to make an accurate diagnosis of schizophrenia. These medical disorders include:

- Infections
- Tumors
- End-stage renal disease
- Hypoglycemia
- Dementias
- Stroke
- Head injuries and
- Vitamin deficiencies, particularly thiamine (vitamin B1)

Drugs Influencing Psychotic Features

- Cannabis (marijuana)
- Amphetamines
- Hallucinogens
- Alcohol and
- Opiates

IS RECOVERY ATTAINABLE IN SCHIZOPHRENIA?

The answer has a lot to do with how recovery is defined. Currently there is no agreed-on definition of recovery pertaining to someone with schizophrenia or a related persistent psychotic disorder. A large part of the current difficulties arise from the lack of precision in some of the terminology, which then creates misunderstanding and unnecessary controversy.

To make matters even more complicated, right now there is no consensus among researchers as to whether schizophrenia is best characterized as a progressive disorder whose natural history is to get worse with time, or a neurodevelopmental problem that, while serious, is not progressive. If the field cannot come to agreement on this issue, this uncertainty creates many challenges in helping clinicians formulate appropriate long-term treatment plans. In spite of these challenges, schizophrenia is treatable with a host of medications, some of which can be used in combination in order to achieve a positive patient outcome.

CHAPTER 4

Depression

Depression is a thief. It robs those affected by it of their capacity to place their values and talents on display. Much like the rhythm of life in general, depression is cyclical for most people who have it—bouts of short-term duration for some, extended duration for others. And then there are those who remain mired in its depths long term—folks on a path of steady deterioration sadly displaying a life not well lived and ending in suicide or some other tragedy. The numbers linked to depression in this country are staggering: Nearly 7 percent of the U.S. adult population—which represents approximately 17.6 million people—is diagnosed with depression, according to the National Institute of Mental Health (NIMH). The National Centers for Disease Control and prevention indicate that depression leads to 200 million lost workdays yearly at an average cost of $30 billion to employers.

Although replete with influences, four factors typically perpetuate depression: social seclusion, poor attitude, gripping fear and a profound feeling of inadequacy, which fuels the belief that one is an imposter who will eventually be "found out" and humiliated. Depression can be a best friend and a safe haven from the perils of the outside world; it can be perceived as something a person can't seem to shake—in spite of their best intentions to do so. It can serve as a source of primary or secondary gain, such as paid leave from work or attracting much desired attention and sympathy.

Assessing these factors thoroughly will be the stepping stones for determining the individual's motivation for getting better. Simply put: <u>the more intimate the relationship with the depression and the greater the gains as a result, the harder it will be to give up.</u>

In the hands of competent clinicians, treatment success rates are quite high. Clinicians emphasizing that the depressed person will have to "action-step" their way out of depression and not just swallow pills serve their clients best. In less competent hands, people will wax and wane symptomatically, never really getting over any humps in a measurable way, and languish.

Many depressed people who enter the treatment system through family practice or primary care fall through the cracks from a management perspective. This occurs for a variety of reasons, with the most common being a lack of both patient and physician follow-up after the initial appointment. It is important therefore, for clinicians to understand the differential diagnosis for this group of clinical syndromes in order to affect positive treatment outcomes.

UNIPOLAR DEPRESSIONS

Unipolar depression, synonymous with the terms *clinical depression* and *major depressive disorder*, is a prolonged state characterized by a group of symptoms that affect thoughts, behavior and feelings and interfere with functioning. These symptoms include persistent sadness or despair, feelings of low self-esteem, apathy, pessimistic thinking, emotional hypersensitivity, irritability, the inability to experience pleasure and thoughts of suicide. Mental health professionals look for a particular combination of symptoms over a significant period of time to arrive at a diagnosis of depression.

It is useful to think of these depressions as "typecast," so to speak. There is the reactive type, the biological type, the mixed type, and an atypical type, to name just a few manifestations.

Reactive depression is a maladaptive response to a specific external event or events. More formally from a DSM perspective, this is an adjustment disorder with depressed mood. Typical examples are difficulty adjusting to a recent divorce, being downsized from a job or the loss of a cherished loved one. Also, there are no measurably significant changes in physical functioning such as sleep patterns, appetite and energy levels with this depression subtype.

Physical depressions—often referred to as biological depressions—on the other hand, typically emerge in the absence of precipitating psychosocial events. Instead, these depressions are endogenous in nature; that is, they "come from within." Biological depressions are associated with physiological changes in bodily systems. They often present with one or more of these core symptoms: change in appetite, change in sleep patterns, psychomotor retardation (thought slowdown accompanied by a decrease in physical movements), anhedonia (the inability to experience pleasure) and decreased libido.

Physical depressions can be medically based. It is hypothesized that certain medical conditions may interfere with neurotransmission in the brain, possibly inhibiting the central nervous system's capacity to get sufficient amounts of the nerve chemicals—norepinephrine, serotonin and dopamine, for example—in the right place at appropriate levels. Diabetes and hypothyroidism are two common culprits influencing depression, with the latter implicated in as many as 10 percent of all severe depressions. In these cases, a thyroid function panel that includes a measure of TSH (thyroid-stimulating hormone) is recommended. Hormonal events can also trigger a biological depression. In women, changes in progestin, estrogen and testosterone levels around the menses can lead to agitation, irritability, insomnia and the possible development of Premenstrual Dysphoric Disorder (PMDD). Low testosterone levels in aging men can cause depression. It is estimated that 20 percent of men between the ages of 60 and 80 have low testosterone levels. Additionally, prescription and recreational drug use can cause chemical changes in the brain resulting in a biological-type depression.

Medical, Drug, and Hormonal Influences on Depression	
Medical Conditions	Autoimmune disorders: AIDS, rheumatoid arthritis, systemic lupus erythematosus, etc. Neurological disorders: Parkinson's disease, etc.
Substance Induced	Prescription medications and recreational drugs.
Hormonal Irregularities	In women: menopause, premenstrual, postpartum. In men: low testosterone in mid to late life.

Mixed depression is a type of depression involving both reactive and biological features. It is a result of brain function that appears to succumb to the effects of psychological stress. When events are extremely stressful, biological changes can occur in the brain, leading to this type of depression. Neither truly exogenous nor endogenous, mixed depressions most likely represent the majority of depressions seen clinically. Typical onset is consistent with the more classic reactive depressions outlined above, but physiological symptoms can develop over time, particularly if the patient does not respond to psychotherapy.

Atypical depression is best thought of as a more severe manifestation of biological depression. The presence of co-existing anxiety disorders seems to be the rule; patients are likely to experience such syndromes as panic disorder and social phobias.

Persistent Depressive Disorder (Dysthymia)

Dysthymia—from the Greek root meaning "bad mind"—is a chronic, low-grade "functional" depression characterized by depressive symptoms that last a minimum of two years in adults and one year in children and adolescents. Symptoms are not absent for more than two months, and they are not caused by a medical condition or the effects of a substance. Those with dysthymia tend to be a uniformly unhappy lot of individuals, yet most of them do not seek treatment. The symptoms are similar to those of major depressive episodes, only milder.

The long-term prevalence of symptom presentation tends to take an exacting toll on the productivity and overall quality of life of people with dysthymia. They are also at high risk for escalation symptoms. As much as 80 percent of people with dysthymia experience at least one episode of major depressive disorder. These more severe episodes, in turn, mask the underlying chronic dysthymic depression. The result is a "double depression."

THE ROLE DRUGS PLAY IN INFLUENCING DEPRESSION

Anti-hypertensives (medications used to treat high blood pressure), anti-Parkinson's agents and beta blockers have been linked to a dysfunctional synthesis of norepinephrine, serotonin and dopamine.

Corticosteroids (including cortisone and prednisone), which some patients take for autoimmune disorders such as systemic lupus and multiple sclerosis, can be problematic too. These can cause not only depression, but even psychotic features. These episodes emerge primarily through high-dose, long-term use.

Alcohol can of course, worsen depression over time. Alcohol activates dopamine receptors in the brain's pleasure center producing a disinhibition effect. Chronic alcohol use though can trigger a phenomenon known as "dopamine receptor down regulation" whereby continued alcohol use produces increasingly diminished reward for the user.

A similar thing can happen to those chronically using benzodiazepines, such as Valium (diazepam), Ativan (lorazepam) and Xanax (alprazolam) for daytime anxiety and insomnia. Benzodiazepines such as these, particularly if used excessively and at doses that exceed the recommended daily maximums, can enhance the actions of GABA only so much before tolerance develops, leading to markedly diminished response rates.

Prescription and Recreational Drugs that Can Cause Depression		
Brand	**Generic**	**Type**
Catapres	clonidine	antihypertensive
Cortone	cortisone acetate	corticosteroid
DepoProvera	medroxyprogesterone	progestin
Dopar	levodopa	anti-parkinson's
Estrace	estradiol	estrogen
Estraderm	estradiol	estrogen
Flagyl	metronidazole	antibiotic; antiparasitic
Inderal	propranolol	beta-blocker
Larodopa	levodopa	anti-parkinson's
Librium	chlordiazepoxide	benzodiazepine
Ogen	estropipate	estrogen
Premarin	conjugated equine estrogens	estrogen
Provera	medroxyprogesterone	progestin
Reglan	metoclopramide	anti-emetic (anti-nausea)
Sinemet	levodopa/carbidopa	anti-parkinson's
Symmetrel	amantadine	anti-parkinson's
Valium	diazepam	benzodiazepine
Xanax	alprazolam	benzodiazepine
		recreational drugs: alcohol amphetamines opiates cocaine marijuana

A New Perspective on Chronic Depression—The Inflammation Model

Although first introduced in the early 1990s, the depression- inflammation connection had not blossomed into something of significance until recently. New clinical thinking is that an inflammatory process is situated "upstream" in the body of a susceptible individual, and that inflammatory "waste" traveling downstream acts as a contaminant which influences the emergence of symptoms we typically ascribe to depression.

The inflammatory model is implicated in conditions such as cardiovascular and autoimmune disorders, diabetes and cancer, so approaching depression as an inflammatory syndrome may open the door to more effective pharmacological interventions capable of delivering results that outshine the paltry track record of antidepressants. Celebrex (celecoxib), an anti-inflammatory, has been found in randomized, placebo-controlled trials to be superior to placebo as an augmenting agent to antidepressants.

The etiology of depression has long been veiled in uncertainty and the likelihood that it is a multifaceted clinical entity with many tentacles attached is becoming more and more plausible. The inflammatory theory may very well prove to be a viable launching pad for the further exploration of more effective treatments for depression; and, together with diet modification, exercise and psychotherapy, anti-inflammatory drugs may reveal themselves to be just the right medicine for targeting depression at its "headwaters."

HOW ABOUT SOME BOTOX FOR DEPRESSION?

Botox, botulinum toxin A, has certainly been on a run in recent years—spreading its wings way beyond its use as an anti-aging treatment. Known primarily for the ability to reduce the appearance of some facial wrinkles, Botox injections are also used to treat such problems as repetitive neck spasms, excessive sweating and overactive bladder. Botox injections may also help prevent chronic migraines in some people.

Now a new study has found that when Botox is injected between the eyebrows, it delivers an antidepressant effect. Researchers at the University of Texas Southwestern conducted a 24-week randomized, double-blind, placebo controlled study that included 30 subjects (93% women in the study) with major depressive disorder. At week 12, the Botox and placebo groups crossed over. That is, those receiving Botox were instead delivered placebo; those getting placebo were then administered Botox.

The subjects who received Botox from the outset or at week 12 had a statistically significant reduction in depressive symptoms compared to those getting placebo. Interestingly, depressive symptoms continued to decline over the full 24-week period after a single Botox injection, while the anti-aging improvements had ceased at the 12–16 week mark.

What's behind Botox's antidepressant properties? We don't know for sure, but it is suspected that Botox's antidepressant effect is "cosmetically" driven, providing an esteem and image boost which in turn improves personal fulfillment. Another possibility is that positive feedback to a happier looking face received from the Botox user's social network provides a sustainable emotional boost. A final suggestion is that the facial muscles communicate with the brain and the act of frowning adversely affects neurotransmission; whereas smiling activates nerve impulses.

CHAPTER 5

Bipolar Disorder

Once devastating and strangely alluring to its sufferers, bipolar disorder was first dubbed "manic-depressive insanity" by 19th century psychiatrist Emil Kraepelin. Today bipolar disorder is characterized mainly by its unpredictable cycle of intense mood swings, typically fluctuating between the two poles of mania and depression.

Bipolar disorder affects approximately 5.7 million adult Americans or about 2.6% of the U.S. population age 18 and older every year, according to the National Institute of Mental Health. Although bipolar disorder affects fewer people than unipolar depression, it can be more destructive to relationships, health, finances and careers. This is due to its related disruptive behaviors, which include delusional thinking, binges and engaging in reckless activities.

More recently referred to as manic-depressive illness, the bipolar spectrum disorders are classified as mood disorders like major depressive illness and dysthymia. All are characterized by a cyclic pattern of mood, behavior and thought processes that fluctuate between mania (or hypomania) and depression.

Mania, according to the current DSM-5, is defined as a "distinct period of abnormally and persistently elevated, expansive, or irritable mood lasting at least one week and present most of the day, nearly every day (or any duration if hospitalization is necessary)." Since mania rarely occurs as a stand-alone clinical condition, its presence usually leads to a bipolar diagnosis.

Hypomania is a mild to moderate level of mania, a period of elevated mood and uncommon energy that lasts at least four consecutive days. It differs from full-blown mania in that symptoms do not cause significant impairment in personal, social or occupational functioning; nor is hospitalization likely to be an issue. Hypomania is often described by patients as pleasurable and exciting, bringing an attendant feeling of enthusiasm and charisma with an apparent free flow of ideas and creativity. Although hypomania may feel

Signs and Symptoms of Manic and Depressive Episodes	
Manic Episode Symptoms:	**Non-manic Bipolar Markers**
Increased energy, activity, restlessness	The patient has had repeated episodes of major depression (four or more, often accompanied by seasonal shifts)
Excessively "high," euphoric mood	The first episode of major depression occurred **before** age 25
Extreme irritability	A **first-degree relative** has a diagnosis of bipolar disorder
Racing thoughts, talking very fast, jumping from one idea to another	When not depressed, mood and energy are a bit higher than average, all the time (**"hyperthymic personality"**)
Distractibility; inability to concentrate; poor judgment; spending sprees	When depressed, **symptoms are "atypical"**: low energy and activity, excessive sleep, profound reactive dysphoria, increased appetite
Unrealistic beliefs in one's abilities and powers	Episodes of major depression are **brief**, less than 3 months
Little sleep needed	The patient has had **psychosis** during an episode of depression
A lasting period of behavior that is different from usual	The patient has had severe **postpartum depression**
Increased sexual drive	The patient has had mania or hypomania while taking an **antidepressant**
Abuse of drugs, particularly cocaine, alcohol and sleeping medications	The patient has had **loss of response** to an antidepressant
Provocative, intrusive or aggressive behavior	**Three or more antidepressants** have been tried, and none have worked
Denial that anything is wrong	
DATA: "Signs and Symptoms of Mania and Depression," National Institute of Mental Health	

satisfying to the person experiencing it, without proper treatment it can escalate into full mania or switch to depression.

Differences between mania and hypomania

Mania:

- Marked occupational and social dysfunction
- Often a need for hospitalization
- 67 percent of patients have a lifetime history of psychosis
- Minimum of one week duration of symptoms according to DSM-5

Hypomania:

- No significant occupational or social dysfunction
- No hospitalization
- No psychotic features
- Minimum four-day symptom duration (average is 2–3 days)
- The pattern of the mood swings determines which of the three types of bipolar disorder is occurring:

Bipolar I: This disorder is characterized by one or more manic or hypomanic episodes with one or more episodes of major depression. In bipolar I, moods can swing dramatically in both directions. The depressions are severe, and the manias may be quite significant in intensity. Episodes of depression in bipolar I must meet the criteria for major depression as outlined in the DSM-5.

Bipolar II: Mood swings involve a severe, full-blown depression as in bipolar I, but the "high" episodes do not reach true mania. This disorder is characterized by the presence of one or more major depressive episodes in combination with at least one episode of hypomania. Bipolar II disorder can be difficult to distinguish from major depression, and at one time the two used to be thought of as variants of the same condition. In fact, the predominant symptomatic presentation is depressive in nature, and an exact definition of what constitutes hypomania can be open to interpretation. Clinicians differ in their capacity and ability to accurately assess it. DSM-5 criteria require that symptoms of hypomania be present for at least four days.

Cyclothymia: This disorder is characterized by mood swings that last for at least two years, with less intense highs and lows than those that occur in bipolar I and II. That is, the episodes do not reach true mania or major depression. However, this can make cyclothymia difficult to diagnose. Cyclothymia is a chronic disorder, and patients typically have a history of numerous hypomanic and depressive episodes. Although characterized by "mild" mood swings, cyclothymia can cause significant distress in daily living due to the abrupt changes from joy to sadness, difficulty sleeping, and problems maintaining the enthusiasm needed to complete projects. Arguably, a diagnosis of cyclothymia may serve as a warning sign of the possible future emergence of a bipolar disorder.

Rapid cycling is defined as a type of bipolar illness in which an individual experiences four or more episodes of mania, hypomania, or major depression within the previous 12- month period. Some individuals cycle from manic episode to manic episode, while others cycle from depressive episode to depressive episode. Still others have mixed episodes that include symptoms of both mania and depression. Episodes can occur over a month, week, or day. Approximately 20 percent of bipolar patients are rapid cyclers; of these, 80 percent are women.

It may be time to reconsider the "phasic" nature of bipolar disorder. A new international study, titled Investigating Manic Phases and Current Trends of Bipolar or IMPACT of Bipolar, found that 64 percent of patients with bipolar I disorder experience symptoms of depression during episodes of mania. As such, depression is of significance during the manic phase of this illness for a considerable number of bipolar I individuals. These findings underscore how nuanced the assessment and diagnosis of bipolar disorder can be and illustrate that bipolarity may not occur in distinct phases as once thought. Therefore treatment considerations, particularly pharmacological ones to be discussed in Chapter 11, should take into account that manic and depressive symptoms mesh with one another and should be managed simultaneously.

Table 5-1 provides a detailed list of the signs and symptoms of mania. However, the seven classic symptoms of mania that deserve the most clinical attention are probably best summed up through the use of the mnemonic:

DIGFAST

Distractibility: Inability to maintain focus on tasks

Insomnia: Reduced need for sleep accompanied by increased energy in spite of little sleep

Grandiosity: Inflated self-esteem

Flight of Ideas: Racing thoughts

Activities: Increase in goal-directed activity—work, social, school

Speech: Excessive, circumstantial, tangential chatter, pressure to keep talking or more talkative than usual

Thoughtlessness: Risky behavior, such as excessive involvement in pleasurable activities that have a significant potential for adverse consequences—excessive spending, risky sexual behavior, reckless driving, gambling, impulsive traveling.

It is essential that the clinician proceed systematically through these seven criteria and ask the client about each one of them, because many will not be volunteered. Ask about past phases in which the client may have experienced a great sense of confidence, an extraordinary feeling of happiness or an uncommon ability to get things done, etc. The next step is to move on to assessing for non-manic symptomology. There are many considerations here, but place emphasis on the following:

- A first-degree relative (mother/father; brother/sister; son/daughter) has a diagnosis of bipolar disorder.
- The first episode of major depressive disorder occurred before the age of 25 (the younger someone is at the first episode, the greater the possibility that bipolar disorder, not unipolar, was the basis for that first episode.
- When depressed, symptoms tend to follow this pattern: very low energy and activity levels; excessive sleeping; increased appetite; increased interpersonal sensitivity to the comments and actions of others; depressive episodes tend to be relatively brief—less than three months in duration.
- Three or more antidepressants have been tried without sufficient response; the individual has experienced mania or hypomania while taking the antidepressant.

Bipolar Symptoms Beyond The DSM

- Ego
- Arrogance
- Entitlement

- Lack of Awareness
- Difficulty Calculating Consequences

Consider Matthew:

Matthew, age 26, was referred to me via the criminal justice system. Matthew was able to successfully hack into his father's IRA account and remove $500,000. Matthew's father had set up simple, easy-to-remember passwords which Matthew easily deciphered. He was able to circumvent other fail-safes, thereby gaining access to the money with which he purchased yet-to-be-developed condo property in South America. Upon discovering this, Matthew's father pressed charges. As a result, Matthew is doing a stint in the New Orleans parish prison system.

The referring judge asked me to evaluate Matthew and make recommendations to the court. As Matthew posed a flight risk, he was accompanied to my office by a court attendant. They arrived early; I had not yet finished up with another client. While waiting, Matthew attempted to pass out his business card to other clients in the waiting room, and this was uncomfortable for these people—to say the least. As I ushered him into my office, he attempted to do the same with me.

Appearing distracted—with pressured speech, flight of ideas and full of grandiosity—our initial session began with him stating that this whole issue over his father's money had been overblown. When I asked why, he said that as an only child, he was going to inherit the money anyway, and since his father is rich, it's no big deal. Because he is in an acutely manic state, he is unable to fathom the gravity of the circumstances he's facing and the seriousness of the potential consequences of his behavior. Matthew's father, supported by his wife, is determined to let the criminal justice system run its course, particularly if Matthew doesn't comply with treatment recommendations.

In Act I, scene 3 of Shakespeare's Hamlet, Polonius speaks these words to his son Laertes: "This above all: to thine own self be true." If you are intolerant of unruly behavior and are easily ruffled by symptom displays like Matthew's, this type of patient will wear you out. So there is nothing wrong with admitting to yourself that you're not personally equipped to best manage such treatment challenges. Instead, keep honing what you are best at instead of laboring to shore up areas where you're not as proficient. Work your strengths and build them big.

Identification and Treatment of Bipolar Disorder is Stuck—Here Is Why:

The major headwinds combating effective identification and treatment include:

- Time from onset of symptoms to accurate identification—if there even is such a thing—can be 10–15 years, because manic symptoms tend to bob and weave and often duck for cover. Mania is hard to recognize when there is considerable time between episodes and the uncooperative nature of affected individuals means they tend not to seek treatment while immersed in the throes of mania.

- Bipolar depressive symptoms are far more prevalent than manic symptoms and thus provide additional cover for mania to hide.

- There is now very credible evidence that 60-plus percent of bipolar I individuals experience symptoms of depression <u>during</u> episodes of mania. Therefore bipolar I and II classifications are time-worn and increasingly irrelevant.

- The etiology of the disorder is quite the conundrum. Excitotoxicity, metabolic issues and neuroplasticity are all parts of the explanatory equation, yet neuroscience is not able to adequately address them so as to have a positive impact on treatment direction.

- There are no animal models with validity. Therefore diagnosis is all over the place.

- The major limitation to novel drug discovery is that there is no consensus on neuropathology, thus pharmacology is all over the place.

- Except for lithium, most treatments for bipolar symptoms were not developed as "anti-polar" therapies (anticonvulsants, second- generation antipsychotics). As such, bipolar disorder has yet to find a good drug fit; the agents readily employed today have been merely repurposed and are best utilized for treating other disorders—physical and mental.

- Even with optimal care, 50 percent of those who achieve symptom remission will relapse within two years. Relapse is influenced by suicide risk and alcohol use. The risk of suicide is highest among all psychiatric disorders at 25 percent. Ditto alcohol problems, which is also at 25 percent.

Because of these headwinds, creativity is all but a must in the treatment and management of bipolar disorder, rendering polypharmacy not only necessary, but also warranted, because of treatment resistance, co-morbidities and substance abuse. Creativity though can open its own can of worms that can crawl all over the bipolar sufferer in the form of intolerable side effects such as weight gain, sedation, malaise, derealization, cognitive fog, new onset type 2 diabetes, hyperlipidemia and hypercholesterolemia.

Irrespective of the treatment modality, outcomes disappoint, so we will have to continue to plow forward and figure out ways to shine more light into the dark spaces of this mystifying mental health condition.

ETIOLOGY

Bipolar disorder is a biologically based illness. Since its first description in 1898, numerous theories have been suggested to explain the disorder's origins. Today, two main approaches are the Kindling Theory and the Catecholamine Theory.

The Kindling Theory hypothesizes that some psychiatric symptoms are a result of biochemical changes in the "emotional brain" that cause nerve cells to become excited. This process causes more neurons to "fire," and the more they fire, the greater the possibility that neurotransmission is going to increase, setting off a constellation of observable and diagnosable symptoms. Left unchecked and untreated, mood fluctuations are likely to occur more often, resulting in the brain becoming increasingly sensitized and the destructive pathways inside the central nervous system being strengthened. According to this theory, a mood disorder is like a fire: Just as a large log burns only with enough time and kindling, so does one unstable mood episode leads to more frequent and more severe episodes in the future.

The Catecholamine Theory suggests that bipolar illness is linked to an increase in cerebrospinal fluid levels of norepinephrine. Catecholamines, such as the naturally occurring chemical compounds norepinephrine and epinephrine (adrenalin), prepare the body for "fight or flight." This theory, proposed by U.S. psychiatrist Joseph Schildkraut, emerged in the 1960s. Schildkraut was particularly interested in norepinephrine. He suggested that a deficiency of this neurotransmitter at receptor sites caused depression, while increased levels caused mania. The Catecholamine Theory demonstrated how pharmacology offered a rational approach to the biology of the brain, and Schildkraut's work is credited with increasing the understanding of the role that biology plays in diagnosing and treating psychiatric illnesses.

OTHER CAUSES

Medical conditions that are linked to increased excitability of neurons can also be associated with mania. These include:

- Central nervous system trauma
- Hyperthyroidism, an endocrine system disorder
- Infectious diseases
- Central nervous system tumors
- Seizure disorders

In addition, certain medications can potentially stimulate neurotransmission of the "emotional chemicals," particularly norepinephrine and dopamine. These medications include:

- Psychostimulants, especially amphetamines
- Antidepressants, especially the cyclics
- The corticosteroid prednisone, in high doses
- Thyroid hormones

SUICIDE

Bipolar patients can be at increased risk for suicide, especially in the earlier stages of the illness. Signs and symptoms to watch for, according to the National Institute of Mental Health, include:

- Talking about feeling suicidal or wanting to die
- Feeling hopeless, believing that nothing will ever change or improve
- Feeling helpless, believing that nothing one does can make a difference
- Feeling like a burden to family and friends
- Abusing alcohol or drugs
- Suddenly putting affairs in order. For example, organizing finances, giving away possessions, etc.
- Writing a suicide note
- Putting oneself in a dangerous situation

Famous People Thought to Have Bipolar Disorder
Ludwig von Beethoven: composer
Russell Brand: actor
Art Buchwald: writer, humorist
Dick Cavett: television personality
Winston Churchill: British prime minister
Vincent van Gogh: artist
Graham Greene: author
George Fredrick Handel: composer
Jimi Hendrix: rock musician
Moss Hart: actor, director, playwright
Vivien Leigh: actress
Gustav Mahler: composer
Sylvia Plath: poet
Edgar Allen Poe: author
Robert Schumann: composer
Britney Spears: pop star
Robert Louis Stevenson: author
August Strindberg: playwright, novelist
Mark Twain: humorist, author
Robin Williams: actor
Virginia Woolf: author

CHAPTER 6

The Many Manifestations of Anxiety

More than 40 million Americans suffer from anxiety disorders, making it the most common mental health complaint in the country. Twice as many women as men experience anxiety disorders. It is unknown, however, whether twice as many women actually suffer from anxiety, or whether they simply are more likely to seek treatment and, therefore be diagnosed. Anxiety manifestations share four common threads: (1) anxiety as a symptom, (2) avoidance as a behavior, (3) fear and (4) threat—whether real or perceived.

Any thorough differential diagnosis of a patient presenting with anxiety symptoms should account for certain general medical conditions, prescription medications and over-the-counter products that may cause, influence or even exacerbate these symptoms. For this reason, a clinician should *never* conclude that a clinical anxiety disorder exists until all possible medical causes have been sufficiently ruled out.

ETIOLOGY

Fight-or-flight is a survival mechanism that has kept the species around for millennia. It is triggered by two closely related chemicals that we have discussed before, norepinephrine and epinephrine. One common depiction of fight-or-flight refers to early man facing a saber-tooth tiger, woolly mammoth or other very real danger of his primitive world. Early man had two choices: He could either confront them (fight) or run from them (flight). Either way, early man's autonomic nervous system prepared physically by dumping noradrenaline, epinephrine and other chemicals into his system. Today, with a dearth of tigers and wooly mammoths in our everyday lives, those stressors have been replaced by events that range from minor aggravations to truly harrowing experiences. Yet the body still reacts the same way it did thousands of years ago.

It is normal to have a fearful reaction when in the presence of actual danger. But an anxiety disorder creates anxiety and panic in the absence of

Other Factors Influencing Anxiety

These medical conditions, prescription- and over-the-counter products are potentially responsible for the emergence of anxiety symptoms.

Medical Conditions

- Angina pectoris: chest pain or discomfort due to coronary heart disease
- Cardiac arrhythmia
- Hypoglycemia: low blood sugar
- Hyperthyroidism
- Premenstrual syndrome

Prescription and Over-the-Counter Products

- Amphetamines, such as Dexedrine (dextroamphetamine) or Ritalin (methylphenidate)
- Appetite suppressants
- Asthma medications, such as Proventil (albuterol), Serevent (salmeterol xinafoate) and Theo-Dur (theophylline)
- Hormone medications, such as oral contraceptives
- Steroids, including prednisone and cortisone
- Nasal decongestants, such as Sudafed (pseudoephedrine)
- Caffeine, found in numerous OTC drugs such as Excedrin, Anacin, No-Doz, Midol and cough remedies; as well as in coffee, tea, caffeinated soft drinks and energy drinks.

actual danger, when the mind is occupied with a possible future danger, or when the reactions are in excess of what most people would experience in similar circumstances. Physical manifestations of anxiety can number in the dozens, and they run the gamut from annoying to frightening. Sweaty palms are one thing; repeated trips to the emergency room, convinced you are having a heart attack, is another,

TYPES OF ANXIETY DISORDERS

Generalized Anxiety Disorder (GAD)

We are all a bit anxious from time to time. The mere stresses of everyday life presents us with situations that we find perplexing and worrisome, igniting the classic fight-or-flight phenomenon. This is consistent with living life on its terms and not ours, that is, none of us really knows what's in store for us on any given day. We can organize ourselves physically and emotionally; we can record a to-do agenda in our physical calendar; we can anticipate potential

---

Symptoms of Anxiety

- Rapid heart rate (tachycardia) or heart pounding
- Palpitations, or feeling of missed heartbeats
- Shallow breathing
- Hand tremors
- Nervousness, muscle tension
- Fingernail biting, picking at skin
- Shortness of breath
- Difficulty concentrating
- Poor attention, "unfocused"
- Easily startled
- Hypervigilance, constantly "on guard"
- Dizziness
- Nausea
- Insomnia
- Diarrhea, frequent urination, or both
- Sweating
- Visual or aural distortions, feelings of unreality

---

roadblocks, interruptions and what might go awry with our day as we have planned it; and still something unexpected, something we have given nary a thought to, pops up and blindsides us as if it came out from the proverbial "left field."

And all of this is okay because it smacks of our having to accept uncertainty and ambiguity as an integral part of getting up every day. And few things are more rewarding than introducing ourselves to an unanticipated challenge, getting acquainted with it, motivating ourselves to go right up to the place where it lives, facing it down and then solving or conquering it. This is the stuff of which self-esteem is made. There is nothing more personally empowering than charting a direction for our lives, plowing through the steps pursuant to reaching our destination and mowing down the inevitable obstacles encountered along the way.

What's happening though to those who fall prey to worrying about the demons that plague their day? The answer is that they are examining what arises in an un-empowered way. The worry consumes a considerable amount of time, and resolved worries are often replaced with new ones. The tail wags the dog, because people cede control to the undesirable problem or nuisance which is driving the worry. And once the worry starts gripping them like a vise, avoidance takes root and little gets accomplished, because solvable obstacles loom as large as King Kong.

Anxiety is as much a cognitive issue as it is an emotional one. Most of us experience anxiety intermittently; it rises to disorder proportions when there is constancy to it. And when chronic, anxiety is invariably linked to faulty, irrational or illogical belief systems which require reframing to make relief attainable.

For people with Generalized Anxiety Disorder, nearly every aspect of life invokes a thought of "what if," leading to a state of chronic worry often accompanied by sensations of doom and gloom. These are folks who: (1) worry all of the time, (2) worry about what they worry about and (3) worry when they're not worrying. This makes GAD a chronic condition, and it is often linked to numerous physical complaints—with headaches, gastrointestinal distress and muscle tension heading the list. It is important to understand that there are positive intentions associated with why people worry. Worrying about something may mean that the worst won't happen, so this is a way of doing justice to a situation fraught with possible negative outcomes.

Specific Phobia

Specific phobias include the fear of dogs, cats, snakes and heights, etc. They are generally not the focus of clinical attention. There is little reason to believe these phobias have a biological basis. As such, people rarely seek either behavioral or medication treatment to manage them.

Social Phobia

Those with social phobia—also known as social anxiety disorder—suffer from an intense fear of doing or saying something that will embarrass them in a public or social setting. Fear of humiliation, rejection and separation may lead them to avoid situations where any of these fears might arise. This results in limiting activities only to those that are known, comfortable or predictable and avoiding any setting that is unfamiliar. This can manifest as a fear, whether of eating in public, attending parties, dating, taking exams, using a public restroom, and public speaking. (Fear of public speaking, in fact, is the number one social fear, shared by an estimated 60 million people.)

These fears can affect many people to varying degrees. These disorders, by contrast, refer to manifestations of social anxiety that rise to levels of clinical significance. They are accompanied by marked impacts on personal, occupational and in particular, social functioning; and they require pharmacologic and non-pharmacologic approaches to treatment.

Panic Disorder

Panic is a brief, intense surge of anxiety, and a panic attack is a period of intense fear or excessive discomfort accompanied by a sensation of immediate danger in situations that may not actually be dangerous. Panic attacks can be debilitating. Symptom presentation may include shortness of breath, palpitations, dizziness, hot flashes or chills, a fear of losing control, even a fear of dying. Symptoms often come "out of the blue," can occur in the absence of obvious stressors and can even occur during sleep. Symptoms last anywhere from a few seconds to several minutes, but the residual effects can linger for several hours.

Panic disorder is usually diagnosed when a person experiences at least four panic attacks in a month, or experiences at least one attack that is accompanied by the fear of future attacks. In other words, attacks rise to disorder proportions when someone hands over control to the panic by worrying excessively about when the next attack will occur and making life changes to avoid them.

Agoraphobia

The literal translation of agoraphobia is "fear of the marketplace," and historically, it has been associated with a fear of open spaces or public places. But today agoraphobia is believed to be a consequence or complication of panic disorder, particularly <u>untreated</u> panic attacks. Approximately one in three people with panic disorder eventually develops agoraphobia, according to the Anxiety Disorders Association of America.

Those with agoraphobia fear experiencing panic-like symptoms in situations where escape may be difficult or embarrassing, or where it may be difficult to obtain help. Such fears can lead to the avoidance of public transportation, automobiles, airplanes, elevators and crowded rooms, etc. In extreme cases, people may stay in their homes for years, fearing that a panic attack would ensue if they were to venture outside their "safe zone."

Adjustment Disorders

These disorders occur in direct response to a specific event or other stressor. Marked distress in excess of what would ordinarily be expected is present, as well as significant impairment in social or other functioning. Once the stressor ends however, the symptoms do not persist for longer than an additional six months. Examples include the termination of a relationship with a significant other, financial difficulties, and marital strife. Adjustment disorder is considered one of the sub-threshold disorders; as such, it is less well defined and can share characteristics of other diagnostic groups. Two common subtypes are adjustment disorder with depressed mood and adjustment disorder with anxiety.

OTHER DISORDERS SEPARATELY CLASSIFIED

Obsessive-Compulsive Disorder (OCD)

In the novel *Moby Dick*, Herman Melville chronicles the obsession that Captain Ahab had with an albino sperm whale that cost him not only a leg, but his life. In the book *Over and Over Again*, authors Fugen Neziroglu and Jose A. Yaryura-Tobias describe OCD as a "full-time companion." Characterized by a series of persistent thoughts and compulsions, OCD is a chronic condition fraught with considerable suffering, shame, guilt and self-doubt. It is often incapacitating, as well. The disorder typically emerges early, often in late childhood, and unfortunately for the affected individual, maintains remarkable symptom stability throughout life.

While most people cling to some habits and routines in their daily lives, for those with OCD, the cycle of repetition can be nothing short of hell on earth. OCD is considered ego-dystonic, meaning most people want to either break or stop the patterns of obsessions and compulsions but find they are unable to do so.

Obsessions are thoughts, images or even ideas that one continues to have over and over again. Common obsessions include a fear of contamination or "germophobia," safety concerns, a need for order or exactness, a fear of evil or sinful thoughts, a constant need for reassurance, and thinking repeatedly about certain words or numbers.

Compulsions by contrast, are ritualistic behaviors or mental exercises performed in response to obsessions. Ostensibly, compulsions reduce the anxiety associated with the obsessions, but this relief is often short- lived. Common compulsive behaviors include:

- **Washing and cleaning.** Repeated washing of the hands.
- **Checking.** Repeated checking of door or window locks, electrical outlets or stove knobs.
- **Ordering and arranging.** A need for symmetry on table tops, with writing instruments or food items in the refrigerator.

- **Hoarding.** The ongoing collection of newspapers, magazines, clothes, canned goods.
- **Mental exercises.** Repeatedly counting or silently stating the same phrase over and over.

As crippling as OCD can be to the individual experiencing it, the effect on their families may be devastating. OCD stirs family conflict, increases angst with regard to how to handle or manage life with the affected individual, and fuels decisions that can lead to separations and divorces.

The etiology of OCD has been controversial and baffling for years. Most experts now believe that OCD is not a result of anxiety, but instead a neurological "short circuit" causing driven, obsessive thoughts and behaviors similar to Body Dysmorphic Disorder, Tourette Syndrome and Hypochondriasis. DSM-5 has removed OCD from the Anxiety Disorders category and placed it in a separate section titled: Obsessive-Compulsive and Related Disorders.

Posttraumatic Stress Disorder (PTSD)

Posttraumatic Stress Disorder has been shifted to a separate section in the DSM-5 titled: Trauma—and Stressor-Related Disorders. This condition is brought on by surviving a severe or unusual psychological or physical trauma. As the name suggests, issues surface after exposure to a real-life traumatic event in which the person believes he or she is in danger and feels extreme fear, horror or helplessness. Historically, PTSD has been considered a disorder most likely to affect soldiers who have been in combat. But in reality, PTSD affects twice as many women as men, according to a recent survey of more than 6,000 American adults.

For example, the lifetime prevalence rates of PTSD for Vietnam veterans and prisoners of war held in World War II are 31 percent and 50 percent, respectively. But for rape victims, the range is 35 percent to 80 percent, according to *The Anxiety Answer Book* by Laurie A. Helgoe, Laura A. Wilhelm, and Martin J. Kommer. Other traumatic events may include childhood sexual or physical abuse, abortion, pregnancy loss, physical attack, being threatened with a weapon, cancer, abusive relationships, auto accidents, fire, and natural disasters such as tornadoes, earthquakes, hurricanes and floods.

Careful study of clinical and biochemical data lead investigators to conclude that PTSD is not a fear- and anxiety-based disorder. Instead, PTSD is one of a wide array of disorders that arise in response to traumatic events. These disorders are characterized by symptoms of avoidance and negative alterations in mood, not fear. They manifest as much more than anxiety.

How Do You Know It Is PTSD?

- A sense of "flashback," feeling as if the initial trauma were happening all over again, with a sense of reliving the event
- Recurring nightmares or daydreams
- Avoiding people, places or things representative of the trauma, including conversations about the event
- Feelings of detachment or estrangement from others
- Intrusive, disturbing memories of the event
- Sleep disturbances
- Angry outbursts
- Hypervigilance, constantly "on guard"
- Disassociation with the event, feelings of "de-realization," a sense that the event did not actually happen

---

Adjustment Disorders

As is the case with PTSD, Adjustment Disorders can be found in the DSM-5 section titled: Trauma—and Stressor-Related Disorders. These disorders occur in direct response to a specific event or other stressor. Marked distress in excess of what would ordinarily be expected is present, as well as significant impairment in social or other functioning. Once the stressor ends however, the symptoms do not persist for longer than an additional six months. Examples include the termination of a relationship with a significant other, financial difficulties, and marital strife. Adjustment disorder is considered one of the sub-threshold disorders; as such, it is less well defined and can share characteristics of other diagnostic groups. Two common subtypes are adjustment disorder with depressed mood and adjustment disorder with anxiety.

Insomnia Disorder

If you believe the media, Americans are in the midst of a sleep-deprivation crisis. Television commercials have displayed everything from Luna Moths entering an open bedroom window to Abe Lincoln and a groundhog reassuring a weary insomniac that his "dreams miss him," and that his sleep problems are treatable. Sleep simply does not come naturally to some people. We're all wired differently and our circadian rhythms are environmentally influenced. And those who travel frequently or do shift work often report difficulties with the sandman.

One estimate puts the cost of sleep deprivation to U.S. businesses at $150 billion a year in absenteeism and lost productivity. There may be something to it. In a recent University of Pennsylvania study, subjects who slept only four to six hours a night for 14 consecutive nights displayed significant deficits in cognitive performance, equivalent to going without sleep for up to three days in a row. The use of sleep agents is quite common and is a boon to the pharmaceutical industry and, if taken responsibly, they can be safe and effective. But they are not the first line of defense when it comes to managing insomnia. Roughly one in four Americans use some form of sleeping pill or other aid in hopes of getting to sleep and staying asleep; and according to BioMarket, a biotech research company, in the year 2004 Americans spent $2 billion on Ambien (zolpidem) alone.

Which of the anxiety and other separately classified disorders discussed above typically respond to medication management? What pharmacological choices are available and how and when are they prescribed? Chapters 12 and 13 will address these questions and also examine other viable treatment alternatives.

SECTION THREE

TREATMENT

CHAPTER 7

Antipsychotics

The modern era for the treatment of the psychotic disorders began in the early 1950s when Thorazine (chlorpromazine) was found to be effective for patients with schizophrenia. Numerous other antipsychotics were then developed and released as treatments for those suffering from psychosis. Today, medication management remains the mainstay of treatment for the psychotic disorders.

HOW ANTIPSYCHOTIC MEDICATIONS WORK

Antipsychotic medications block dopamine receptors in the central nervous system. The blocking actions on dopamine receptors in the limbic system are thought to underlie the effectiveness of these agents in managing the "positive" symptoms of schizophrenia. However, because of their actions on a number of neurotransmitter systems, a veritable host of side effects may emerge. These are powerful drugs, and like all medications, they have both

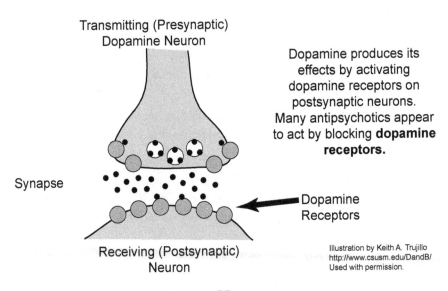

Transmitting (Presynaptic) Dopamine Neuron

Dopamine produces its effects by activating dopamine receptors on postsynaptic neurons. Many antipsychotics appear to act by blocking **dopamine receptors.**

Synapse

Dopamine Receptors

Receiving (Postsynaptic) Neuron

Illustration by Keith A. Trujillo
http://www.csusm.edu/DandB/
Used with permission.

55

benefits and risks. When these drugs are effective, the patient feels more relaxed, less fearful, more confident and better able to concentrate. Thought distortion, mood and sleep patterns may also improve. Antipsychotics may or may not be sedating, depending on product selection. Antipsychotic medications fall into two main categories: the older conventional agents and the newer atypical agents.

Conventional Agents

The first antipsychotic to emerge on the U.S. drug market was Thorazine (chlorpromazine) in 1952. Others followed, including Haldol (haloperidol), Navane (thiothixene) and Stelazine (trifluperazine). Today, these first-generation medications are no longer considered the agents of choice for treating psychotic manifestations, having given way over the past several years to the newer atypical or second-generation antipsychotics. All of these first-generation agents are effective in treating mania but ineffective in managing bipolar depression. Conventional antipsychotics fell out of favor due to pivotal shortcomings—two in particular. First, they are responsible for a group of neurological adverse events known as extrapyramidal symptoms (EPS). Second, approximately 20 percent of adults with schizophrenia are unresponsive to conventional antipsychotics.

Side Effects of the Conventional Agents   As stated earlier, extrapyramidal symptoms are a cluster of neurological adverse effects of antipsychotic drugs, and they are common with the use of the conventional agents. Those occurring most often include:

> **Dystonia:** The most common manifestation of EPS, it is characterized by muscle-tightening in the neck and shoulders, accompanied by spasms.
>
> **Parkinsonian:** Produces muscle rigidity, mask-like facies, tremor, shuffling gait and diminished arm-swing.
>
> **Akathisia:** This type of EPS is characterized by motor-restlessness, a need to move and an inability to sit still.
>
> **Tardive dyskinesia:** Though not a type of EPS, it is a most feared adverse effect. It is characterized by involuntary facial movements involving the tongue, eyes, lips and face. Tardive dyskinesia is generally associated with long-term use of conventional

antipsychotics. Once present, it is considered irreversible, although some patients show a slow remission of symptoms over time.

When an EPS manifestation develops, one treatment is to lower the dosage of the offending drug. But pharmacological treatments can also be utilized. Agents such as Benadryl (diphenhydramine) and Cogentin (benztropine) can be administered either orally or intramuscularly. Other side effects of the conventional agents may include:

- Dry mouth, blurred vision, constipation, sedation and memory problems Orthostatic hypotension—a drop in standing blood pressure
- Weight gain, particularly with Thorazine (chlorpromazine)
- Grand mal seizures
- Increased levels of prolactin (a hormone related to growth hormone) and
- Neuroleptic malignant syndrome

Atypical Antipsychotic Agents

Over the past 25 years, a new generation of agents has emerged. These so-called atypical or second-generation medications were developed to meet the treatment needs of those unresponsive to the conventional agents and to improve the overall tolerability of antipsychotic use.

The term "atypical" helps differentiate these antipsychotics from the older, conventional ones. More important, however, is that the atypicals are not a single, homogeneous class of drugs. Instead, they differ from one another with respect to receptor affinity, effectiveness and side effects. Because their blocking actions of dopamine (D2) postsynaptic receptors vary, and collectively these drugs are strong serotonin (5-HT2A) blockers, they carry a lower risk of extrapyramidal side effects and tardive dyskinesia. All of the atypicals are approved for the treatment of bipolar mania. However, effectiveness varies considerably from patient to patient, depending on symptomatic circumstances. Currently, there are ten atypical antipsychotics available on the U.S. drug market:

Clozaril (clozapine): Introduced in 1990, this was the first of the atypical medications and has been referred to as a miracle for otherwise treatment-resistant patients. Clozaril is the prototype to this day, considered to be the most effective, but also the most dangerous.

Clozaril: A Double-Edged Sword
Clozaril (clozapine) was introduced in the United States in 1990, after being used in Europe since the 1970s. Although this drug has been extremely successful in treating schizophrenia, it also carries more than its share of risks. For this reason, it is not a first-line drug of choice, and careful monitoring is necessary.

Benefits:

- "Gold standard" effectiveness compared to other antipsychotics
- Some improvement in cognitive function
- Effective in decreasing hallucinations and delusions
- FDA-approved for the treatment of recurrent suicidal behavior
- Can help with smoking cessation in some patients
- Can diminish symptoms of aggression and violence
- Can decrease alcohol use in patients who abuse alcohol
- Very low incidence of EPS and akathisia and
- Almost no tardive dyskinesia

Risks:

- May cause agranulocytosis, a potentially fatal decrease in white blood cell count that can subject a patient to opportunistic infection
- Blood work (particularly white blood cell (WBC) counts) are mandated by the FDA according to established guidelines (weekly for six months, although after this period, monitoring can then take place on a biweekly basis)
- Can interact with other drugs that also decrease WBC count, such as Tegretol (carbamazepine) and some antibiotics
- Some deaths have been reported, due to myocarditis, an inflammation or degeneration of the heart muscle
- Over-sedation
- Major weight gain
- Elevated risk of Type 2 diabetes and potential for increasing triglycerides and cholesterol
- Can cause urinary incontinence
- Seizures at higher doses are common (greater than 600mg/day) and
- May take many weeks, even months, to be effective

Risperdal (risperidone): In addition to its formidable track record as an antipsychotic, this medication is well-accepted for the treatment of agitation and aggression in dementia, in spite of a "black box" warning. It is FDA approved for minimizing temper tantrums, aggression and self-injury associated with autism, as well as disruptive behavior disorders in children and adolescents (ages 5–16). Risperdal (risperidone) gained FDA approval in 2007 for the treatment of schizophrenia in adolescents ages 13 to 17. The drug has few side effects at lower dosing ranges (below 6mg/day). Above 6mg/day, EPS symptoms are a concern. It is available in a long acting injectable formulation named Risperdal Consta (risperidone microspheres IM).

Zyprexa (olanzapine): Zyprexa provides rapid calming action for agitation associated with schizophrenia. The drug is rather sedating and likely produces the most weight gain among the antipsychotics. Like Clozaril, it too is linked to an increased risk of Type 2 diabetes as well as elevated triglyceride and cholesterol levels—all of which may potentially be significant. Zyprexa benefits from having a low discontinuation rate among its users. It is available as an extended-release injectable suspension which goes by the brand name Relprevv (olanzapine pamoate).

Seroquel (quetiapine): Studies support the use of this drug for the management of aggressive, cognitive and affective symptoms of schizophrenia. Seroquel (quetiapine) and its extended-release companion Seroquel XR (quetiapine extended-release) are FDA-approved for bipolar depression. There is essentially no EPS or tardive dyskinesia with this medication. In recent years for better or worse, it has been increasingly prescribed as a sleeping pill. Seroquel (quetiapine) has demonstrated abuse potential, particularly when crushed and snorted via the intranasal route or crushed, liquefied and then injected intravenously.

Geodon (ziprasidone): This is the least likely of the atypicals to cause weight gain, and it is also the least sedating. Its pharmacological profile suggests potential advantages for associated anxiety and depression, although the drug is associated with agitation at lower doses. But because Geodon (ziprasidone) has been linked to cases of fatal cardiac arrhythmia, it is not a first-line treatment of choice. For this reason, a thorough cardiac work-up is recommended before use. Geodon (ziprasidone) is available as an intramuscular injection.

Abilify (aripiprazole): Abilify (aripiprazole) is becoming fairly well established as an effective treatment for a number of disorders.

It is FDA-approved as an augmenting agent in treatment-resistant unipolar depression and is increasingly being employed as augmentation to the selective serotonin reuptake inhibitors (SSRIs) when managing resistant obsessive-compulsive disorder (OCD). Abilify (aripiprazole) is associated with minimal weight gain and sedation and has few other side effects. One potential disadvantage is that Abilify (aripiprazole) is not sedating enough to effectively manage acute agitation.

Invega (paliperidone): Invega (paliperidone) is actually an active metabolite of Risperdal (risperidone)—note the similarity in their generic names. Because its delivery system to the bloodstream allows for extended action (24 hours), it can be dosed once daily. Reputable clinical studies indicate that Invega (paliperidone) has no clear therapeutic advantages over Risperidal (risperidone) or, for that matter, the other atypicals. Similar to Geodon (ziprasidone), it also carries some cardiac risk and is metabolized primarily by the kidneys, so it is not associated with as many potential drug interactions nor does it need dosage adjustment in patients with liver disease. It is available as an injectable—Invega Sustenna (paliperidone palmitate).

Fanapt (iloperidone): After receiving a "Not Approvable" letter from the FDA in July, 2008, Vanda Pharmaceuticals gained FDA approval for this medication in May, 2009. Fanapt (iloperidone) was actually 15 years in the making, and its ownership has been handed off back and forth among several companies likely due to suboptimal efficacy. And Fanapt's (iloperidone) less than impressive efficacy is not helped by its side effect profile. This drug must be titrated up slowly to minimize orthostatic hypotension and dizziness. Start at 1 mg twice daily, increasing by no more than 2 mg per day over the next week to reach the target dose range of 12–24 mg/day. Cardiac effects appear to be similar to those of Geodon (ziprasidone). This medication's checkered track record precludes it from being considered a first-line antipsychotic agent.

Saphris (asenapine): Saphris (asenapine) was FDA approved in August, 2009. It is available only as a sublingual tablet so therefore not a prescribing clinician's first choice, because oral second-generation agents remain the favored route of administration. Saphris (asenapine) is significant for weight gain but does not rival

Zyprexa (olanzapine) in this category. Because it is administered sublingually, oral numbness can be a problem. Like Fanapt (iloperidone), Saphris (asenapine) has not distinguished itself so as to be considered a first-line choice.

Latuda (lurasidone): The most recent entry running in the second-generation antipsychotic derby is Latuda (lurasidone). It is the tenth atypical antipsychotic on the U.S. drug market. The drug-maker Sunovion Pharmaceuticals announced FDA approval in October 2010. Latuda (lurasidone) causes very little weight gain but is significant for sedation. Metabolic syndrome effects (Type 2 diabetes, elevated triglyceride and cholesterol levels) are minimal. Latuda (lurasidone) is indicated for the treatment of schizophrenia in adults and for treatment of major depressive episodes associated with bipolar I disorder (bipolar depression) as monotherapy and as adjunctive therapy with lithium or valproate. This drug seems to work as well as the other major atypical players. It is very expensive though (as are the other patent-protected agents) with an average dosing regimen pricing out at $5000 or more per year.

Side Effects of the Atypical Agents   In general, the side effects of the atypical agents are more benign than those of the older, conventional agents. As mentioned previously, there is less EPS and a lower risk of tardive dyskinesia. The most common side effects of the atypicals are weight gain, sedation, insomnia, agitation, constipation and dry mouth.

However, as mentioned above in their respective sections, both Clozaril (clozapine) and Zyprexa (olanzapine) have been linked to a significantly increased risk of Type II diabetes and an additional risk of increasing triglyceride and cholesterol levels. Collectively, these risks are referred to as "metabolic syndrome." All of the atypicals are associated with metabolic syndrome to some extent. However, Geodon (ziprasidone) and Abilify (aripiprazole) have minimal metabolic risks and therefore stand out in this regard. Metabolic effects have yet to be adequately established for the agents discussed above that have more recently come to the U.S. market.

Overall effective treatment of schizophrenia from a symptom domain perspective continues to be elusive. Reliable, valid studies fail to demonstrate that negative symptoms and cognitive problems are responding sufficiently to any of our present medications, creating a genuine dilemma for both clinicians and patients.

ANTIPSYCHOTIC RISK WHEN USED IN DEMENTIA

Antipsychotics are often used in dementia patients with associated symptoms of agitation, irritability and disruptive behavior; although the FDA, several years ago, issued a black-box warning outlining an increased risk of sudden death when used in this special population group.

The risk of death in dementia patients utilizing antipsychotics varies rather widely, depending on the agent employed, according to a study published online in the British Medical Journal in late February, 2012. The study examined 75,000 nursing home patients (a large sample size) with dementia for risk of possible death within six months of the initiation of antipsychotic medication. The study looked at Haldol (haloperidol), Seroquel (quetiapine) and Risperdal (risperidone), in particular.

Patients placed on Haldol (haloperidone) demonstrated a doubling in their risk of mortality compared with those placed on Risperdal (risperidone)— while Seroquel (quetiapine) users were significantly less likely to expire compared to the Risperdal (risperidone) users. Seroquel (quetiapine), although seemingly safer than others in this sample, didn't work as well in dementia patients. This finding is not surprising. I have taught that Risperdal (risperidone) is the agent of choice within the 2nd generation antipsychotic group for years now in my Psychopharmacology seminars. This does not mean that Risperdal (risperidone) is devoid of risk, but at a low dose (less than 1 or 2 mg per day) the drug has minimal side effects; whereas Haldol (haloperidol) is prone to cause extrapyramidal symptoms, thereby exacerbating agitation and disruptive behavioral sequences in these patients. Nondrug intervention strategies should always be utilized first in elderly dementia patients.

UNAPPROVED USE OF ANTIPSYCHOTICS: AN EVER-GROWING CONCERN

In 1996, the three second-generation antipsychotics FDA approved at that time—Clozaril (clozapine), Risperdal (risperidone) and Zyprexa (olanzapine)—were prescribed for patients with anxiety disorders in 10 percent of office visits. The bulk of the prescribing for anxiety was with Risperdal (risperidone) and Zyprexa (olanzapine) because Clozaril (clozapine) was not—and still is not—considered a first-line agent of choice due to potentially serious concerns with agranulocytosis. A decade later, in 2006, prescribing had more than doubled for the treatment of anxiety despite absolutely no evidence that antipsychotics are effective for anxiety disorders and clear evidence that this psychotropic class is associated with severe and even life-threatening side effects. And this mass over-prescribing was done off-label, mind you. Atypical antipsychotics have clawed their way along to $15 billion in sales per year despite the fact that much of the prescribing is unsupported by scientific evidence, lacks clear rationale, and is bringing obesity and its attendant risks more to the problematic forefront.

As alarming as the potential consequences of overuse may be, it is not really surprising. A few so-called psychiatric "thought leaders" have been working in concert with pharmaceutical companies to promote off-label use of these agents for years now. And they are succeeding because the use of these drugs is indicative of a lack of caution that now permeates everyday prescribing practices.

This is not an indictment of this psychotropic medication class. Used appropriately, antipsychotics are a godsend to the management of the psychotic spectrum disorders. In fact, acute psychotic features could not be managed effectively without them. But there is no justification for the fact that objective sales data indicate they have become pharmaceutical best-sellers. They shouldn't be.

COGNITIVE-BEHAVIORAL AND FAMILY THERAPY FOR SCHIZOPHRENIA AS AN ADJUNCT TO ANTIPSYCHOTIC MANAGEMENT

Cognitive-behavioral treatment (CBT) for the psychotic spectrum—schizophrenia in particular—is quite similar approach-wise to what would be employed for depression or anxiety. But CBT for schizophrenia also addresses issues more relevant to the psychotic features themselves such as positive and negative symptoms as well as overall life management.

Over 90 studies regarding the efficacy of CBT for schizophrenia have been conducted; sample sizes however, are on the small side. The conclusion to be drawn is that CBT appears to be most effective for positive symptoms (delusions, hallucinations, exaggerated, disorganized speech and behavior) and is a suggested treatment in the American Psychiatric Association practice guidelines. Here's an example: when it comes to hallucinations, the psychotherapist could suggest that the affected person try to increase the volume of the voices he is hearing—attempt to make them louder and more belligerent-sounding. The goal is that if the person insisted that he had no control over the voices and is then able to tell the therapist that he was able to make the voices louder and more vocal, the professional could then say "well if you can make them louder and more intense, let's try to make them softer and less volatile."

Treating negative symptoms (loss of pleasure, emotional withdrawal, passivity, apathy) with CBT is similar to behavioral interventions utilized in depression. Getting them moving and avoiding social isolation are key steps. People with schizophrenia are no different from healthy subjects when it comes to how they view pleasure. Inertia sets in when thoughts about pleasure don't square with actually experiencing something pleasurable. So CBT is built around teaching them not to downplay the fun and enjoyment associated with getting together with friends in their thoughts before actually going out and finding how enjoyable it turned out to be.

CBT and medication management work hand-in- hand. CBT can serve as a tool for patients who are medication non-compliant by helping them chart their symptoms, and if uncontrollable, realize that medication may be worth a try.

Multifamily work involves bringing together several families, including the identified patients, for what amounts to an educational get-together. This family-style intervention may run for up to a year and typically consists of bimonthly sessions. The focus of this work is on simple problem solving. Basically one problem is selected for the group to work on with family members from the different groups drawing on the social support of each other. Ideas about how to solve commonly shared problems are exchanged and solutions are reached. For example, an issue that may be discussed is how to encourage the affected individual to develop and maintain a routine.

Families reach a consensus that this begins with getting out of bed at a regular time each morning, then grooming oneself, eating breakfast and deciding on the steps to be stressed for maintaining structure for the rest of the day. Less is more here while the individual is in a fragile state of learning, and families learn from each other how much to push patients toward desired behaviors, and possibly invite disobedience versus when to back off. Also, families are taught how to recognize the prodromal, or early warning signs of symptom return with emphasis placed on contacting the treating professional(s) promptly—if or when this occurs.

What You, Your Clients and Family Members Need to Know

Relapse is common in schizophrenia due to noncompliance with medications. With those affected by schizophrenia or any other chronic psychotic spectrum disorder, typically two things happen: First, these folks take their medications, start to feel better, and then stop, believing they are "cured." Second, patients in the throes of a psychotic episode can be convinced that the medications are really a poison or a form of mind control. The patient's family is often in a position to observe the prodromal symptoms—early warning signs of possible symptomatic resumption—so involving the family in discussions about the significant benefits of medication compliance can be important and helpful.

CASE STUDY: SCHIZOPHRENIA—"THE VOICES WERE TELLING ME"

Leonard is a 22-year-old homeless man who was recently arrested for bathing nude in a fountain adjacent to an upscale hotel. The police have transported Leonard to a private psychiatric facility at which you are a clinical social worker, and his case is referred to you. It is difficult to obtain a clear history from Leonard, because he rambles incessantly, often changing the subject while making bizarre and incoherent statements. He is able to report, however, that during the last month he has been generally unable to sleep, and that when he did sleep, he often experienced what he calls "strange dreams." Leonard appears emaciated and reeks of alcohol. When asked about his arrest, Leonard states that he simply found the hotel fountain a convenient location for a bath.

Leonard admits to hearing voices over the past few weeks, and he reports that on the day he was arrested, the voices were telling him to "be sure to bathe the feet of all the passers-by, because this was Holy Week." He explains that he was just getting ready to do that when "someone from the hotel reported me."

Because of Leonard's indigent status, your facility's case management department asks you to refer Leonard to a state-operated psychiatric hospital. After a consultation with a psychiatrist at the state facility, you are made aware that Leonard is well known to the staff. The psychiatrist mentions that Leonard is routinely treated with psychiatric medication, and that upon symptom remission, he is released. The doctor adds that numerous attempts to locate any of Leonard's family members or friends have failed, as have all attempts to locate placement for him, because "he doesn't follow the rules." The doctor concludes by saying that Leonard is one of the facility's many "revolving door" patients that they expect to see repeatedly over time.

DIAGNOSTIC CONSIDERATIONS

Given that Leonard is well known to the staff at the state psychiatric facility, he had previously been diagnosed with chronic paranoid schizophrenia. Leonard's psychotic symptoms improved on Risperdal (risperidone) in the past, so the attending psychiatrist decided to begin with 2 mg (in divided doses) on day one of treatment. The dosing regimen was increased by 2 mg per day to a total daily dose of 8 mg over a four-day course of administration.

TREATMENT COURSE

Leonard remained in the hospital for another three days and then was discharged on 8 mg of Risperdal (risperidone) per day after demonstrating much symptom improvement. Leonard's prognosis for maintaining symptom remission was poor, however, given his tendencies toward medication non-compliance after getting better and his decision to remain homeless.

Dosage Range Chart—Antipsychotic Medications

Brand Name	Generic Name	Class	Daily Dosage Range*
Abilify	aripiprazole	atypical	10mg–30mg
Clozaril	clozapine	atypical	300mg–600mg
Fanapt	iloperidone	atypical	12mg–24mg
Geodon	ziprasidone	atypical	120mg–160mg
Haldol	haloperidol	conventional	1mg–40mg
Invega	paliperidone	atypical	3mg–12mg
Latuda	lurasidone	atypical	40mg–120mg
Mellaril	thioridazine	conventional	150mg–800mg
Moban	molindone	conventional	20mg–225mg
Navane	thiothixene	conventional	10mg–60mg
Prolixin	fluphenazine	conventional	3mg–45mg
Risperdal	risperidone	atypical	4mg–16mg
Saphris	asenapine	atypical	10mg–20mg
Seroquel	quetiapine	atypical	300mg–600mg
Stelazine	trifluoperazine	conventional	2mg–40mg
Thorazine	chlorpromazine	conventional	60mg–800mg
Zyprexa	olanzapine	atypical	5mg–20mg

* Suggested adult dose
Note: Dosage ranges may vary depending on source, and may also vary according to age.

CHAPTER 8

Antidepressants

In 1990, Prozac (fluoxetine) became the first drug to be featured on the cover of a major U.S. news magazine, marked a turning point in pharmaceutical history. Prozac (fluoxetine), hailed as a "miracle" drug of sorts, was introduced in the United States in 1988. Two years later it was the most widely prescribed drug in this country, earning a place as *Newsweek*'s "cover drug" with the headline "Prozac: A Breakthrough Drug for Depression."

Prozac may have emerged as a 20th century star, but many of its predecessors had long been utilized in managing not only unipolar depression, but also bipolar depression, obsessive compulsive disorder, social anxiety disorder, substance abuse syndromes, panic disorder, eating disorders, premenstrual disorders and anxiety disorders.

HOW ANTIDEPRESSANTS WORK

A primary role of medication is to attempt to restore normal biological functioning. For antidepressants, the location of that functioning resides in the 100 billion nerve cells that are contained within the human brain. The nervous system depends on communication among these many nerve cells.

THE STRUCTURE

A nerve cell consists of a cell body, dendrites, an axon and a terminal. Each *cell body* manufactures its own messenger molecules, more typically referred to as neurotransmitters. For the sake of this discussion, these are norepinephrine, serotonin, dopamine and GABA.

Dendrites are structures shaped like tree branches that fan out from the cell body. They accept and send information to the cell body, serving as a message exchange system that facilitates intracellular communication.

Axons are fibrous tubes that serve to transmit impulses away from the cell body. After the neurotransmitters are manufactured, they travel along this tube-like passageway away from the body of the cell. Then they are stored within small "sacs" or vesicles within the presynaptic terminal.

THE PROCESS

One of the films in the famous Star Wars trilogy was *The Empire Strikes Back*. Keep this in mind as we embark upon my story of: *Serotonin and the Synaptic Sea*.

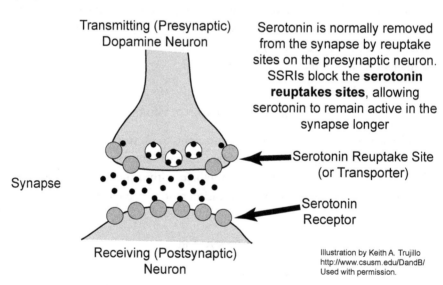

Transmitting (Presynaptic) Dopamine Neuron

Serotonin is normally removed from the synapse by reuptake sites on the presynaptic neuron. SSRIs block the **serotonin reuptakes sites**, allowing serotonin to remain active in the synapse longer

Serotonin Reuptake Site (or Transporter)

Synapse

Serotonin Receptor

Receiving (Postsynaptic) Neuron

Illustration by Keith A. Trujillo
http://www.csusm.edu/DandB/
Used with permission.

Serotonin is the neurochemical most often implicated in mood regulation. Cell bodies within our brains make it for us, and after it is manufactured, to do us any good, it has to get somewhere. But first, it has to get moving. Pushed by a wave of chemical and electrical impulses, it travels through a fibrous tube (axon) and is deposited in little storage tanks (pre-synaptic vesicles) before its real work begins. Its journey begins when these storage tanks dump it into the synaptic sea (synaptic cleft). It then sails the synaptic sea in search of docking stations (post-synaptic receptors). Serotonin's appointed duty is to influence these tiny proteins (receptors) by activating them or inhibiting them. After doing so, it is transported back (reuptake) for repackaging and is recycled, awaiting another journey.

This is the natural order of the biochemical process associated with mood regulation for all of us. And it doesn't like to be messed with. Let me explain: Approximately 10 percent of the adult population uses antidepressants, and their use in children and adolescents is increasing at a substantial rate. With this in mind, let's harken back to our little serotonin fable above. An antidepressant's primary role is to block the reuptake of serotonin into pre-synaptic cells forcing this neurotransmitter to remain in the synaptic sea longer. I'm sure you get the "drift" here. The longer serotonin can remain in the synaptic cleft, the greater the possibility it can do its thing at the docking stations (receptors). Sounds good in theory, but multiple bodies of well-respected clinical work tell us that the Empire (brain) doesn't take too kindly to such manipulation. And as such, it strikes back. Here's how: perturbed by this artificial manipulation, the brain undergoes a series of compensatory mechanisms in an effort to maintain the normal functioning sequence outlined earlier. To get a little fancier, the brain seeks to restore its "homeostatic balance" or equilibrium. (There is nothing at all unusual about this; every system in the universe seeks to do the same thing after getting out of kilter for a while.) And here is what the brain does: armed with feedback forces, presynaptic nerve cells begin releasing less serotonin than usual, and in lockstep, the density level of the docking stations (post-synaptic receptors) diminishes. In simple terms, there are less of them. So as the antidepressant tries to continue accelerating serotonin activity, the brain responds by putting the hammer down. Wanna guess who wins?

The takeaway here: On-going use of an antidepressant may promote diminishing returns. In the early 1990s, only 10–15 percent of people with major depression progressed to chronicity—becoming treatment-resistant. Today, 40 percent or more are treatment-resistant. Coincidentally, SSRI use exploded from the early 1990s to present. To make matters worse, this compensatory process often develops in people who had a satisfactory initial response to an antidepressant, and therefore continued to take the drug. Eighty percent of those maintained on an antidepressant experience symptom re-occurrence, and the longer people use them the greater the risk of relapse. So through treatment, they get worse.

For years now, I have been reporting in my blog space and in my seminars that the vast majority of my patients using antidepressants report a "plateauing" effect, particularly those using these agents for mild to moderate depression or dysthymia—for which they are not indicated! And my concern through these many years has been that persistent use promotes resistance. Antidepressants are to mental health medicine what antibiotics are to physical medicine when it comes to overuse. More is not more, so it is best that antidepressant users realign their expectations, and that prescribers reinforce the limitations of these drugs when it comes to what users want from them. Think months of use—not years.

To resurrect the tagline from a popular 1970s TV commercial for Chiffon margarine, "**It's not nice to fool Mother Nature!**"

Antidepressants—An Initial Look

Anyone contemplating the use of an antidepressant should first ask themselves: a) what do I want the drug to do? b) for how long? Antidepressants are prescribed in droves, often cavalierly, for the wrong symptom set with few questions asked. Rates of antidepressant use continue to rise with 11 percent of the general population now taking these medications. Benign signs of depression and intermittent anxiety associated with the ups and downs of everyday life yield prescriptions in all but a heartbeat nowadays. Then users hitch their wagons to these drugs only to be disappointed because of faulty expectations. The faultiest of expectations regarding antidepressants is that these drugs will fill some kind of happiness or contentment void. They don't, and that is displeasure just waiting in the wings. Another faulty outlook is that these drugs will somehow change behavior—rescuing the user from having to do the often painstakingly hard work of identifying the who's, what's, where's when's and how's contributing to or driving their discontent. In my experience, expectations are often skewed among those who shouldn't have been prescribed antidepressants in the first place; whereas the severely depressed often view these drugs as an opportunity to get a leg up, which is quite reasonable.

Many people begin antidepressant use with a sort of blind faith, attributing power to these drugs to change troubling circumstances for the better—power antidepressants don't have. Nor are these people getting the straight scoop on what to expect, particularly from the media. Television, internet and print ads paint a picture which amounts to little more than false hope. The television commercials in particular, speak the language the consumer can accommodate, and the compassionate, caring voiceover frames the drug as the pathway to relief. They have enormous appeal to a population of depressed people intent on getting a quick fix and instant gratification. Impressionable people are exposed to antidepressant ads claiming that "simple pleasures shouldn't hurt," others show folks happily dancing in lily fields purportedly resulting from antidepressant use. These ads are enormously powerful and play directly to the consumer's perceived vulnerabilities. The technology revolution has us all buying. So with the aid of their healthcare providers, consumers should commit themselves to understanding the limitations of these agents. They are not the singular solution to depression woes. Otherwise, they will fall prey to media claims that can accurately be described as antidepressant overreach.

Types of Antidepressants

- Cyclics
- Selective serotonin reuptake inhibitors (SSRIs)
- Serotonin and norepinephrine reuptake inhibitors (SNRIs)
- Norepinephrine reuptake inhibitors (NRIs)
- Monoamine oxidase inhibitors (MAOIs)
- Atypical antidepressants
- Hybrids

Cyclics

Also referred to as tricyclics, these are among the oldest group of antidepressants, dating from the 1950s. One of the very first cyclics, Tofranil (imipramine), was originally developed as an antispychotic, but was subsequently found to possess antidepressant properties. Other cyclics include Elavil (amitriptyline), Anafranil (clomipramine) and Desyrel (trazodone). Many of these agents are dual-action in that they block the reuptake of both serotonin and norepinephrine.

Elavil (amitriptyline) has an established efficacy in the management of chronic pain. For years, Anafranil (clomipramine) was the drug of choice in the treatment of obsessive-compulsive disorder, but it was eventually supplanted by the selective serotonin reuptake inhibitors. Desyrel (trazodone) has proven to be quite effective in the management of depression associated with concomitant anxiety and insomnia.

The cyclics are indeed effective antidepressants. In fact, they were preferred treatments from the 1950s to the 1990s. Unfortunately, the cyclics are fraught with side effects that render them intolerable for many patients:

- As a class, they tend to be dangerous in overdose and can enhance the sedative effects of alcohol.
- They are sedating, in that they inhibit the effects of histamine, similar to the actions of Benadryl (diphenhydramine).

- They can cause annoying side effects—such as dry mouth, blurred vision, constipation, urinary retention and confusion—because they block the actions of the neurotransmitter acetylcholine.

- They can cause orthostatic hypotension, a drop in standing blood pressure.

- There is a risk of tachycardia, or rapid heart rate.

- Weight gain is associated with a metabolic slowdown in carbohydrate and fat metabolism. In some individuals, weight gain is contributed to by an increased craving for sweets and fats.

- A decrease in libido and an inability to perform sexually is linked to the serotonergic effects of these antidepressants.

Selective Serotonin Reuptake Inhibitors (SSRIs)

The SSRIs are indeed popular—one of the most famous ending up on the cover of *Newsweek* magazine, as noted above. Prozac (fluoxetine) was the first of a new class of drugs called selective serotonin reuptake inhibitors (SSRIs) that went on to become the most prescribed class of antidepressants. By today's treatment standards, approximately 70 percent of all new antidepressant prescriptions are for an SSRI.

These medications work by selectively blocking or inhibiting the reuptake of the neurotransmitter serotonin. In addition to Prozac, other SSRIs include Sarafem (fluoxetine, like Prozac); Zoloft (sertraline); Paxil (paroxetine); Celexa (citalopram); Lexapro (escitalopram); Luvox (fluvoxamine) and Brintellix (vortioxetine).

As a class, the SSRIs are better tolerated than the cyclics. They have the advantage of once-a-day dosing and are much safer in overdose than the cyclic agents. There is, however, insufficient data to support the efficacy of SSRIs over the cyclic antidepressants.

Side effects of the SSRIs tend to be related to an increase in serotonin activity, and they tend to be fewer than those of the older cyclic antidepressants. SSRI side effects also tend to be transient, with the exception of weight gain and sexual dysfunction, which are associated with long-term use. The main side effects include:

- Increased anxiety or an "activated" feeling

- Sedation

- Insomnia

- Sexual dysfunction

•Weight gain, but less than that associated with older antidepressants. One study noted an average weight gain of four pounds over a six-month period.

Discontinuing SSRIs is best done gradually to spare patients unnecessary upset. Abruptly stopping an SSRI is linked to a withdrawal syndrome in which some patients report "electric shock sensations" in the hands and feet accompanied by painful "brain zaps" in the head. Although unpleasant, these effects are not considered dangerous to either the brain or the extremities.

Serotonin and Norepinephrine Reuptake Inhibitors (SNRIs)

SNRIs are considered dual-action antidepressants. That is, they inhibit or block the reuptake of both serotonin and norepinephrine. The model drug in this category is Effexor (venlafaxine). This drug was marketed as "Prozac with a punch." The "punch" refers to Effexor's (venlafaxine) effect on norepinephrine. At doses of less than 150 mg, Effexor (venlafaxine) is essentially no different than a typical SSRI. But at doses of 150 mg or higher, Effexor (venlafaxine) is said to block the reuptake of serotonin and norepinephrine. Cymbalta (duloxetine) is approved for the treatment of major depressive disorder and diabetic neuropathic pain. It is also demonstrating promising results in the management of chronic pain and stress urinary incontinence.

Effexor (venlafaxine) may cause high blood pressure, especially at doses of 225 mg per day or higher. Patients taking Effexor (venlafaxine) at these doses are encouraged to monitor their blood pressure at least once per day. The effects of Cymbalta (duloxetine) on blood pressure are not well established. Otherwise, the side effects of the SNRIs are similar to those of the SSRIs.

Another SNRI is Pristiq (desvenlafaxine). Faced with the fact that the Wyeth drug company (at the time) was losing patent protection for its top-selling antidepressant Effexor XR (venlafaxine XR), the company needed a brand product that would potentially replace some of the revenue loss when Effexor XR (venlafaxine XR) went generic in 2010. Sales of Effexor XR (venlafaxine XR) in 2007 hovered around 3.8 billion dollars. Wyeth claimed that Pristiq (desvenlafaxine) had distinct advantages over Effexor XR (venlafaxine XR). Among them were that patients could begin taking Pristiq (desvenlafaxine) at the therapeutic dose of 50 milligrams daily thereby circumventing the "start low, go slow" gradual increases associated with determining the appropriate dose for the user. Another advantage of Pristiq (desvenlafaxine) according to Dr. Philip Ninan, a Wyeth vice president for neuroscience, was that Pristiq (desvenlafaxine) was unlikely to interact with other medications metabolized by the liver.

But several analysts were skeptical of Pristiq (desvenlafaxine) claiming that it had not set itself apart from other antidepressants on the market, and that its market release appeared primarily to have the drug serve as a "patent extender" for Effexor XR (venlafaxine XR). This is because Pristiq (desvenlafaxine) is a primary active metabolite of Effexor (venlafaxine) meaning Pristiq (desvenlafaxine) is the chemical compound that results after Effexor (venlafaxine) is taken, metabolized and processed by the body. The most commonly reported side effect of Pristiq (desvenlafaxine) is nausea. Also, blood pressure needs to be monitored.

In July of 2013, the FDA approved a new serotonin norepinephrine reuptake inhibitor (SNRI), Fetzima (levomilnacipran) for major depressive disorder (MDD) in adults only. The efficacy of Fetzima (levomilnacipran) at once-daily doses of 40–120mg was established in three randomized, placebo-controlled studies in adults with MDD. Fetzima (levomilnacipran) is essentially an isomer—a clone, so to speak—of the SNRI Savella (milnacipran), which is approved for the treatment of fibromyalgia. The interesting thing here is that Fetzima (levomilnacipran) is not approved for fibromyalgia and Savella (milnacipran) is not approved for depression. Go figure. The side effects of Fetzima (levomilnacipran) are the usual suspects—nausea, increased heart rate, palpitations, erectile dysfunction and other associated SNRI side effects. There's nothing new here, merely another makeover for treating depression.

Norepinephrine Reuptake Inhibitors (NRIs)

The antidepressant Strattera (atomoxetine) selectively blocks the reuptake of norepinephrine. Strattera (atomoxetine) is FDA-approved for the treatment of ADHD. Although pharmacologically considered an antidepressant, it is not FDA-approved for the treatment of depression. NRIs are noted for providing an energy boost, as well as for decreasing distractibility and improving attention span.

Monoamine Oxidase Inhibitors (MAOIs)

Monoamine oxidase inhibitors (MAOIs) were first developed in the 1950s and today are rarely used, due to their numerous and potentially serious drug-drug interactions and drug-food interactions.

Monoamine oxidase is an enzyme that circulates in the central nervous system to metabolize neurotransmitters at presynaptic nerve endings. The antidepressant properties of the MAOIs are linked to the fact that these agents inhibit the actions of this enzyme. Two common MAOIs are Parnate (tranylcypromine) and Nardil (phenelzine).

A monoamine oxidase inhibitor transdermal delivery system (patch) called Emsam (selegiline) is also available. Pharmacokinetically, the patch

Food Products that Contain Tyramine

Because of potentially serious drug-food interactions—for example, a sudden, dangerous spike in blood pressure—the following foods should be avoided while taking monoamine oxidase inhibitor drugs (MAOIs). This is *not* a complete list, and patients should consult their physicians.

Alcohol
> Beer and ale (including non-alcoholic varieties), red wine, port, whiskey, liqueurs, vermouth, sherry, Riesling, sauternes.

Aged cheeses
> American, blue, Boursault, brie, camembert, cheddar, Roquefort, Stilton, Swiss, parmesan, processed, mozzarella, gruyere, Romano

Fish
> Smoked, pickled, dried or fermented. This list includes herring and fish roe, such as caviar.

Aged or cured meats
> Including sausages, bologna, salami, pepperoni, game meats and canned meats

Meat tenderizer, meat extracts

Fermented bean curd products
> tofu, miso soup

Fava beans

Fruits and vegetables
> Overripe avocados and figs; raisins, bananas, red plums, tomatoes, spinach and eggplant

Sour cream, yogurt

Sauerkraut

Shrimp paste

Brewer's yeast or yeast extracts

Powdered and liquid protein dietary supplements

Vitamins and supplements containing yeast

delivers its active ingredient by way of absorption through the skin. Purportedly, this delivery system is associated with fewer side effects when compared with the oral administration of the MAOIs.

MAOIs are linked to a host of drug-drug interactions. For example, an extremely dangerous and possibly fatal interaction may occur when Demerol (meperidine) is combined with an MAOI. Patients taking an MAOI also need to be cautioned about the use of over-the-counter drugs, such as the common cough remedy dextromethorpan.

Potentially serious drug-food interactions also make the MAOIs problematic. Tyramine is an amino acid that plays a role in maintaining blood pressure and is metabolized by monoamine oxidase. Foods containing tyramine, if combined with MAOIs, can result in a hypertensive crisis as arterial blood pressure rises, at times suddenly. Patients should be provided with a list of tyramine-containing foods to avoid while taking MAOIs. Also, MAOIs should never be combined with SSRIs for fear of the development of "serotonin syndrome." Characterized by fever, profuse sweating, rigidity, twitching, rapid pulse, high blood pressure, confusion and altered consciousness, serotonin syndrome can result in a coma or even death.

Atypical Antidepressants

Atypicals don't fit specifically into an antidepressant "family" as the others do. In this category, the antidepressant of note is Wellbutrin (bupropion). This medication's efficacy is likely linked to its action on dopamine and norepinephrine nerve cells. It can be considered a dopamine and norepinephrine reuptake inhibitor (DNRI). Some studies suggest that Wellbutrin (bupropion) does not destabilize the moods of bipolar patients, resulting in fewer of them tipping into mania or rapid cycling.

The primary side effects of Wellbutrin (bupropion) are anxiety and insomnia. The insomnia can be significant to the point of requiring management with a prescription hypnotic (sleep-aid). Wellbutrin (bupropion) is associated with few, if any, sexual side effects. But there is a seizure risk at doses greater than 400 mg a day, which is why it is contraindicated in seizure disorder. This medication is also contraindicated in alcohol withdrawal, since that condition can lead to seizures, as is also the case in patients with eating disorders.

Zyban (bupropion) is a slow-release form of Wellbutrin (bupropion) that has been approved by the FDA as a treatment for smoking cessation. A dosage of 150 mg twice daily is recommended to help people abstain from smoking and avoid subsequent weight gain.

Aplenzin (bupropion hydrobromide), was approved by the FDA in April 2008. Sanofi-Aventis U.S. markets the product in the United States and Puerto Rico. The Aplenzin (bupropion hydrobromide) 522 mg dose is the only FDA-approved single-tablet, once daily treatment equivalent to 450 mg of Wellbutrin (bupropion) therapy.

Oleptro, (trazodone extended-release), approved by the FDA in February 2010, is a long-acting offspring of the popular immediate-release antidepressant trazodone. Oleptro (trazodone extended-release) sports a combination of rapid and sustained-release technology that claims to maintain blood levels within therapeutic range for 24 hours, potentially reducing the incidence and severity of side effects while maintaining efficacy in the treatment of major depressive disorder in adults.

Remeron (mirtazapine) works indirectly on norepinephrine and serotonin as did Serzone (nefazodone) before it was removed from the U.S. drug market by its manufacturer Bristol-Meyers Squibb in June, 2004. Serzone (nefazodone) was linked to dozens of liver failures in Europe, Australia, New Zealand and Canada, and was taken off those markets prior to its removal in the United States. The generic formulation (nefazodone) remains available, however, in the U.S.

Remeron (mirtazapine) seems to help with the anxiety and sleep problems common to depression. With Remeron (mirtazapine) however, weight gain due to an increase in appetite is very common. In rare instances, Remeron (mirtazapine) also decreases white blood-cell count.

Hybrid Antidepressants

Viibryd (vilazodone) combines the mechanism of action of SSRIs like Prozac (fluoxetine) and Lexapro (escitalopram) with that of the anti-anxiety drug Buspar (buspirone)—which targets a specific serotonin receptor, 5-HT1A. (Buspar is discussed later in this book). If this drug's brand name sounds as though it may be somewhat of a "hybrid" antidepressant, you are right. Viibryd (vilazodone) is not another "me-too;" it exerts a dual-action effect on the neurotransmitter serotonin by inhibiting serotonin reuptake as the SSRIs do, and by acting as a partial agonist at the 5-HT1A serotonin receptor. This antidepressant seems promising, but time will tell. Also, its dual-action effect does not mean the drug will outperform other serotonin agents. Viibryd (vilazodone) is reportedly associated with minimal weight gain and fewer sexual side effects.

Enter Brintellix (vortioxetine) for depression. It received FDA approval in September, 2013. This approval comes on the heels of the FDA giving the green light to Fetzima (levomilnacipran) in July 2013—which I've written about in the SNRI section above. Like the SSRIs, Brintellix (vortioxetine) is a serotonin reuptake inhibitor. It's also an activator of the serotonin receptor subtype, 5HT1A, mentioned in relationship to Viibryd (vilazodone) in the section directly above. So, is this essentially another Viibryd (vilazodone)? I would say yes. There are some receptor binding differences between these two, but receptor binding capabilities are often overrated and denote advantages that are mostly theoretical in nature. Translation: Don't view a drug's chemistry as gospel for providing the intended effect. Brintellix's (vortioxetine) approval was based on the usual and customary placebo studies which revealed that the effective dosage range of this drug is from 5mg to 20mg daily. As for side effects, nausea was the most commonly reported adverse event, while weight gain was negligible.

INITIATING ANTIDEPRESSANT SELECTION: WHAT'S IMPORTANT

It is certainly important to know whether the antidepressant consistently outperforms placebo—based on well-designed, clinically relevant studies—for what's being treated. Another factor is how well the antidepressant stands up to other competitors within the same genre. When it comes to employing antidepressants, there is no clear cut right way or wrong way. There are only possibilities.

> **How the depression presents.** There are several subtypes of major depressive disorder, but none of them are reliable predictors of antidepressant response. Nevertheless, there needs to be a starting point for the selection process. For example, is the client's depression accompanied by anxiety and insomnia, or is it characterized by melancholia, hypersomnia and a vegetative state? In the first example, any of the SSRIs with the likely exception of Prozac (fluoxetine) because of its energizing properties, would be acceptable choices; the latter example would be better served by Prozac (fluoxetine), the SNRIs (Effexor (venlafaxine), Cymbalta (duloxetine), Pristiq (desvenlafaxine) etc.) or Wellbutrin (bupropion).
>
> **Personal and family history.** Has the client had any previous experience with an antidepressant? If yes, what were the results? If the medication was discontinued, why? If it worked, try it again, unless the client's clinical condition has changed enough to no longer warrant its use. Does the client's history include a family member who was prescribed an antidepressant drug and responded to it favorably? If so, use this possible DNA phenomenon to the client's advantage by using the same medication.
>
> **Drug characteristics.** Prozac (fluoxetine) and Wellbutrin (bupropion) are examples of "energizing" antidepressants; whereas Paxil (paroxetine) and Celexa (citalopram) tend to be more sedating. Initial choices therefore, should be predicated on how the depression presents—as outlined in #2 above. The point here is that one size does not fit all, and selection should not be based on what samples are in abundant supply or what pharmaceutical representative just visited.
>
> **Reasonable expectations.** When anyone is started on an antidepressant, the individual should be informed as to what to expect from the

drug. Inform them that antidepressants may take several weeks to generate any consistently noticeable mood improvement. They should be counseled to take the medication as prescribed for a defined period of time—say six months—before a reassessment.

Initial response. This one's important. After the first swallow, and with some waxing and waning for at least a few days, there will be side effects. Side effects tend to annoy patients, so when in a vulnerable state, it's easy for them to give up. If you believe the person may be at risk for non-compliance or stopping the medication altogether, some cheerleading may be necessary because the most critical phase of antidepressant management is the first 7–10 days of treatment. Encourage patients to stay with the drug because many side effects will abate within a week of antidepressant initiation. (Not all side effects, for sure. Physiological adverse events such as sexual dysfunction may persist for some time.)

Let the client choose. Initial antidepressant selection is solely within the prescriber's domain, right? Not so fast. No one antidepressant or antidepressant class consistently outperforms another. So let the client choose his or her antidepressant based on acceptable side effects. By acceptable side effects, I mean those that the client is willing to put up with or tolerate. Prepare your client for an antidepressant trial by <u>first</u> focusing on the drug's side effects—not therapeutic effects. Then have them share their selections with the prescriber, where they are not likely to get much pushback—unless there are threatening contraindications. Proceeding in this manner helps the client put side effects in perspective, which in turn tends to mitigate the annoyance of having to endure them in the first place. Also, getting the client involved in the selection process has them believing they have "skin in the game" when it comes to what they will be taking. The result: exercisable choices fuel empowerment and empowerment fuels compliance. That's win-win. Finally, finding the right antidepressant fit can be tedious. Users should enlist the support of trusted family, friends and maybe even colleagues for encouragement as needed.

Handling Medication Side Effects

In a "perfect drug" scenario, medications would zero in on their intended target systems producing only desired, therapeutic effects then metabolize and leave the body. Unfortunately it's not that simple, as medications act in a scatter-shot sort of way by finding unintended receptor targets—producing adverse, unwanted and undesirable effects as well.

You must be honest with clients about medication side effects and this issue should be discussed up front, preferably before medication initiation. Point out that although practically every drug—prescription and over-the-counter—has side effects, many of them are short-lived and "run their course" as the body gradually adapts to the new substance. Then discuss them, focusing only on those most frequently reported. Keep it simple.

You might also want to suggest ways for combating certain side effects. For example, medications that are linked to the adverse effects of anxiety and insomnia are best taken in the morning. More sedating medications should be taken at bedtime; those associated with nausea should be taken with food.

There are instances where the side effects of antidepressants can be an advantage to treatment. Getting depressed people moving is essential. It's even more essential for those spending inordinate amounts of time in bed, cutting themselves off from social contact with others. Melancholic, vegetative depressions can be a long slow slog, particularly if motivation for improvement is low. So for the patient intent on getting better, but who is also listless, lethargic and socially isolated, the activating side effects of certain antidepressants can be a plus. The goal would be to disrupt the unhealthy equilibrium to which the individual has fallen prey, assuming compliance with the medication regimen. Activating antidepressants like Prozac (fluoxetine), the SNRIs and Wellbutrin (bupropion) can be rather stimulating. Users may report feeling hyperexcited and anxious. It's important not to view these effects as counterproductive to treatment, but instead as a vehicle for changing inertia into energy to get the person moving! Disrupting the behavioral status quo produces "dis" ease that can influence the emergence of positive behavioral steps such as getting out of bed, getting to the breakfast table, attention to personal hygiene and even venturing out for a walk or a visit to a local coffee shop—initial steps that are critical to longer-term, more sustained improvement.

MANAGING ANTIDEPRESSANT-INDUCED SEXUAL DYSFUNCTION

Ironic isn't it? Depression robs people of their desire for sex, and antidepressants can make the situation even worse. Sexual dysfunction, which includes diminished libido, decrease in arousal and/or vaginal dryness for women and erectile dysfunction in men, is common in both genders with depression. And although this is bad enough, antidepressant use delivers a double whammy.

On average, 50 percent of men and women who use antidepressant medications such as the SSRIs and SNRIs experience sexual difficulties. Fortunately there are ways to manage this issue that you may wish to discuss with your clients in cooperation with their physician or other prescriber:

Consider medical possibilities first. The initial step should be to consider the possibility of medical causes for the sexual dysfunction. A number of physical illnesses are linked to low libido, a decrease in pleasure and performance difficulties. Hormonal irregularities such as estrogen imbalance in women and low testosterone counts in men may also be culprits. Doctors and other prescribers can order any number of tests to determine if these issues apply.

Don't abruptly discontinue. Antidepressant use should never be stopped without consulting the prescriber. Reclaiming sexual intimacy is not a worthwhile trade-off if the depression returns, because the cycle will start all over again.

Dosage Reduction. Again, in conjunction with the prescriber, it may be possible to reduce the antidepressant dose sufficiently enough to mitigate sexual side effects while still obtaining depression relief. And gradual dosage reduction is a goal worth pursuing anyway as depressive symptoms improve.

Take the antidepressant after sexual activity. It is very possible that the daily dose can be scheduled soon after the time the client would ordinarily engage in sexual activity. This is when blood levels of the drug would be at their lowest. For example, if sexual intimacy usually occurs at night, the dose can be taken right after sex.

Medications that treat sexual dysfunction. Drugs indicated for erectile dysfunction, such as Viagra, may be helpful in men and even women. Clients should not try this without medical consultation and supervision. Viagra can be potentially dangerous, particularly in those who take nitrates for certain heart conditions.

Drug holidays. Clients can discuss the option of taking breaks from their medication. By taking a periodic two-day respite from antidepressants, the rate and incidence of sexual side effects can be lowered without markedly increasing the risk of relapse.

Switch to an antidepressant that typically causes fewer sexual side effects. The antidepressant Wellbutrin (bupropion HCL) has consistently been shown to have less of an effect on sexual function compared to other agents such as Prozac (fluoxetine), Zoloft (sertraline), Lexapro (escitalopram) and Effexor (venlafaxine). But the benefits of switching to offset sexual difficulties must be carefully weighed against the possibility that Wellbutrin (bupropion HCL) may not be as effective for managing the depression. Give it a fair trial and take a "wait-and-see" approach.

Augmentation. Sometimes simply adding Wellbutrin (bupropion HCL) to an antidepressant that is linked to sexual dysfunction can make a difference. The advantage of this option is that sexual performance improves somewhat, and the use of two agents reinforces the possibility of sustained symptom improvement.

By following these suggestions, most men and women can achieve reasonably satisfying sexual intimacy while using antidepressants. These medications don't have to infringe upon an otherwise satisfying love life.

ANTIDEPRESSANT EFFECTS ON SLEEP

Cyclic antidepressants. The cyclic antidepressants have long been associated with managing insomnia associated with depression. Most of these agents are sedating and suppress REM sleep. The sedating cyclics typically block the actions of serotonin and histamine, examples include Elavil (amitriptyline) and doxepin. Doxepin is sold here in the U.S. under the brand name Silenor, in 3mg and 6mg strengths for primary insomnia. In recent years, treating clinicians have come to understand the importance of scaling back the dosages of these antidepressants to avoid daytime drowsiness and sleepiness.

Desyrel (trazodone) and its first cousin Serzone (nefazodone) do not suppress REM, although the latter has fallen out of favor due to liver toxicity which in some instances resulted in fatalities. Because trazodone does not markedly affect REM, it remains a favorite on most formularies. Doses in the 50mg to 100mg range nightly are generally sufficient.

SSRIs. When it comes to sleep, the regulation of serotonin is complicated due to the quantity and quality of serotonin receptor activity. Prozac (fluoxetine) and Paxil (paroxetine) have been studied the most, but as a class, the SSRIs appear to slow the onset of sleep and increase the number of awakenings—leading to an overall poor sleep cycle. Also, the SSRIs suppress REM sleep and are linked to intense and vivid dreams.

SNRIs. Not surprisingly this group, including the agents Effexor (venlafaxine), Cymbalta (duloxetine) and Pristiq (desvenlafaxine) is reported to have effects on sleep that are similar to the SSRIs. Sleep continuity and REM are compromised by these antidepressants and their norepinephrine activating effects are unfriendly to sleep initiation and continuation.

Atypicals. The atypical antidepressant Remeron (mirtazapine) possesses the three-fold action of norepinephrine, serotonin and histamine inhibition and blockade. The drug's profile therefore provides a strong basis for helping users get to sleep quickly and stay asleep longer. In fact, some users sleep too much—up to 12 hours per day. Daytime somnolence can be a problem and Remeron (mirtazapine) produces the most weight gain among all of the contemporary antidepressants. A dosing range of 7.5mg to 30mg nightly is sufficient.

Wellbutrin (bupropion HCL) differs from all of the other agents discussed in that it has no serotonin effects. Although Wellbutrin (bupropion HCL) does not suppress REM sleep, increased activation of norepinephrine and dopamine often leads to complaints of insomnia, particularly difficulty getting to sleep.

Knowledge of how different antidepressants affect the sleep spectrum is an important determinant when it comes to selecting an agent that most suitably meets the needs of depressed patients.

Do Antidepressants Really Deliver?

In one widely-reported meta-analysis, a researcher dismissed antidepressant efficacy in all but the most severe cases of depression. Then another research team tackled the very same data and reached a very different conclusion: antidepressants are effective in all but the <u>mildest</u> cases of depression. If you were to read only the abstracts of these works, it would be reasonable to think that these different conclusions represent solely the biases of the respective authors. Further examination of each body of work however, indicates that different statistical methodology was employed in each, and therefore such details could influence different conclusions. This is the conundrum when it comes to statistical research. Outcomes are linked to whom you ask and the parameters of the statistical methods. So the devil is indeed in the details.

Another issue is the process of patient selection. Those selected for clinical trials are hardly representative of outpatients as we tend to think of them. Patient selection typically excludes those with previous suicide attempts and bipolar, psychotic, co-occurring medical illness, substance abuse and personality disorder issues. In the real world of clinical practice, co-morbidity is the rule, not the exception. Thus applying results from efficacy studies conducted in a much more "sterile" manner to real-life situations is nonsensical. Another issue is that of study dropouts. When side effect-influenced dropouts are excluded from outcomes data, positive outcomes for antidepressants are inflated. Another strike against design methodology.

Putting all of these factors together, it comes down to this: Approximately a quarter of those treated with one antidepressant medication realize a full remission of symptoms. Those remaining (three quarters of users) continue to exhibit subclinical symptoms which linger on long-term. All of this goes to show how extraordinarily complex clinical depression is, underscoring the importance of having a bevy of diverse, yet complementary approaches for treating it.

Some Final Takeaways on Antidepressants

The cultural bar for what is considered depression is getting lower and lower. Thus, antidepressants are being increasingly prescribed for the wrong symptom set—psychosocial stress is not an indication for use. Long-term use of these drugs fuels "oppositional tolerance" as well as antidepressant-induced tardive dysphoria and some 73 percent of improvement with antidepressants is now attributed to the placebo effect. A trial of antidepressants has been successful when:

The user begins feeling more energetic, brighter and motivated after several days of use.

The energy and motivation boost propel the user to act in her best interest—goal setting, organizing herself personally and professionally, chipping away day-to-day at what she wants to accomplish, ramped-up social interaction, improved attitude and facing her fears rather than succumbing to them.

The user concluded from day 1 that use should be time-limited and that the drug had no magical powers to solve her problems, unilaterally change her behavior or do the work only she could do for what she wants to master.

Most importantly, the user thought through the process of antidepressant use, understanding their benefits and limitations and didn't subscribe to false hope.

CASE STUDY: DEPRESSION—"I JUST DON'T HAVE ANY ENERGY LATELY"

Rhetta is a 25-year-old woman who presents to her family practitioner for her annual physical examination and Pap smear. She is a single heterosexual female, a vegetarian who does not drink alcohol or smoke, and tests negative for substance abuse. She is currently taking Lo-Ovral-28, an oral contraceptive, one tablet daily. She relates a 14-pound weight loss in the last two months. She also complains of a lack of energy, but she has trouble falling asleep. She works part-time as a youth director at a local church while pursuing a master's degree in art at a local university. She complains of the stress generated by her demanding job and attending school at the same time. She has had considerable difficulty concentrating over the past four weeks and has not turned in a class project that was due last week. Being a talented artist, some of her work has been on display at statewide festivals and exhibits. Presently, however, she expresses little interest in painting and is thinking about leaving graduate school. Rhetta is the youngest of four siblings, with alcoholic parents. When she was eight years old, her mother died of liver cirrhosis. She was placed in foster care in the fourth grade. An older sister is taking Zoloft (sertraline) for depression.

Rhetta is appropriately dressed with clean clothes. She sobs at times during the interview. Her affect is sad, her mood is depressed, and she admits to having suicidal ideation but no specific plan. She is oriented to person, place, and time, but she displays some recent memory deficits accompanied by poor concentration. She is of above average intelligence with satisfactory insight and judgment, and she denies hearing voices or having other hallucinations.

DIAGNOSTIC CONSIDERATIONS

Rhetta's treating physician concludes that she is experiencing a major depressive episode. Though this depression seems to have developed due to her difficulty in adjusting to work and school demands, symptomatically she is experiencing physiological symptoms as well. As a result, her doctor recommends she try an antidepressant. She agrees to do so and is started on Zoloft (sertraline), 25 mg daily for one week, then increasing to 50 mg daily for one week, and then 100 mg daily thereafter. The physician explains the common side effects associated with Zoloft (sertraline), that it may take three to four weeks for symptoms to improve, and that she should do her best to not miss any doses. He also mentions that since she has a sister taking Zoloft (sertraline), it may prove to be a good choice for her also.

TREATMENT COURSE

Rhetta responds favorably to this Zoloft (sertraline) regimen. Although she does experience some of the side effects her doctor mentioned, they are manageable. After six weeks, many of the clinical depression symptoms have abated, although she reports still not feeling enthusiastic about her life. (This is a common subclinical, residual symptom of depression). She is instructed to remain on the Zoloft (sertraline) for another three months and to then schedule a follow-up appointment for re-evaluation.

Dosage Range Chart—Antidepressants

Brand Name	Generic Name	class	Daily Dosage Range*
Anafranil	clomipramine	cyclic	150mg–250mg
Aplenzin	bupropion (Hbr)	atypical	174mg–522mg
Brintellix	vortioxetine	hybrid	10mg–20mg
Celexa	citalopram	SSRI	20mg–80mg
Cymbalta	duloxetine	SNRI	20mg–80mg
Desyrel	trazodone	cyclic	150mg–400mg
Effexor	venlafaxine	SNRI	75mg–350mg
Effexor XR	venlafaxine XR	SNRI	75mg–350mg
Elavil	amitriptyline	cyclic	100mg–300mg
Emsam (patch)	selegiline	MAOI	6mg–12mg
Fetzima	levomilnacipran	SNRI	40mg–120mg
Lexapro	escitalopram	SSRI	10mg–40mg
Luvox	fluvoxamine	SSRI	100mg–400mg
Nardil	phenelzine	MAOI	45mg–60mg
Nefazodone (Serzone)	generic only	atypical	100mg–500mg
Norpramin	desipramine	cyclic	150mg–300mg
Oleptro	trazodone extended	cyclic	150mg–300mg
Pamelor	nortriptyline	cyclic	75mg–150mg
Parnate	tranylcypromine	MAOI	20mg–60mg
Paxil	paroxetine	SSRI	20mg–50mg
Pristiq	desvenlafaxine	SNRI	50mg–100mg
Prozac	fluoxetine	SSRI	20mg–80mg
Remeron	mirtazapine	atypical	15mg–45mg
Sarafem	fluoxetine	SSRI	20mg–80mg
Sinequan	doxepin	cyclic	150mg–300mg
Strattera	atomoxetine	NRI	60mg–120mg
Symbyax	olanzapine/fluoxetine	atypical	6mg olanz/25mg fluox
Tofranil	imipramine	cyclic	150mg–300mg
Viibryd	vilazodone	SSRI/atypical	10mg–40mg
Wellbutrin SR	bupropion (sustained)	atypical	150mg–300mg
Wellbutrin XL	bupropion (extended)	atypical	150mg–300mg
Zoloft	sertraline	SSRI	50mg–200mg

* Suggested adult dose

Note: Dosage ranges may vary depending on source, and may vary according to age.

CHAPTER 9

Treatment-Resistant Depression

Treatment-resistant depression (TRD) is exactly what it sounds like—a depression that is mostly or partially resistant to treatment. One definition of TRD is a depression that has failed to respond to a course of treatment over a minimum of four to six weeks of two or more antidepressants. Some estimates place this at 40–60 percent of all cases of depression.

The need for viable augmentation strategies to assist in the pharmacological management of treatment-resistant depression (TRD) has become so dire that clinicians seem to perk up to any option nowadays. This is understandable given the rather paltry track record linked to traditional antidepressants when used as monotherapy in the treatment of depression.

The genesis of treatment-resistant depression is linked to how neurotransmitters are born. Cell bodies manufacture their own messenger molecules—more typically referred to as neurotransmitters. The neurotransmitters thought to play the biggest role in mood stability— norepinephrine, serotonin and dopamine—are generated via pathways that start with amino acids and end with the neurotransmitters just mentioned. The problem is that we humans are not all able to manufacture the same amount of neurotransmitters. Our individual rate of development also varies and is controlled by our genotype. Since antidepressants don't aid in the actual manufacturing of these messenger molecules and are not genotype-specific, remission rates among those using these medications are quite variable. Widespread clinical evidence from multiple, well-respected sources spells out the following: Only 30 percent of depressed subjects achieve remission on their first antidepressant trial; subsequent trials yield only a 40–50 percent symptom remission rate. With remission rates as low as they are, treating clinicians are increasingly drawn to additive medication strategies that will hopefully lead to clinical improvement for their patients.

Research into the efficacy of treating depression via the use of one antidepressant alone—known as monotherapy—continues to raise a specter of doubt. The most sobering statistics regarding TRD come from the National Institute of Mental Health:

- 55 percent to 65 percent of depressed subjects utilizing one antidepressant alone demonstrate a partial or even no response.
- 35 percent to 45 percent do enter into active remission, but of these, one quarter to one third of these subjects continue to display residual symptoms of depression.

Conclusion: Monotherapy is not adequate for most depressed subjects, particularly long term.

PHARMACOLOGICAL AUGMENTATION STRATEGIES FOR TREATING TRD

Augmentation refers to the addition of medication from different chemical classes or the combination of antidepressants. The goal of any augmentation treatment strategy is to enhance the actions of norepinephrine, serotonin, dopamine and even GABA enough to facilitate mood improvement.

Additive Strategies

Lithium: The addition of lithium to the treatment regimens of nonresponsive patients has been investigated in repeated controlled studies. It is frequently the first-choice treatment for patients who have failed to respond or have only partially responded to antidepressant monotherapy. Don't underestimate lithium's efficacy as a "kick-starter" when combined with the SSRIs in particular.

Thyroid Supplements: Because adequate thyroid function is so important to metabolism and mood, adding thyroid supplements such as Synthroid and Levothroid (both T4), and/or Cytomel (T3), may prove beneficial. Subclinical thyroid function is often linked to poor antidepressant response, and thyroid-stimulating hormone (TSH) levels which are elevated but still within the normal range of 2.0 – 3.0 may contribute to compromised antidepressant response. The best case scenario for those meeting DSM-5 criteria for Major Depressive Disorder would be to get TSH levels in the 1.0 range. For those with TSH levels only slightly above normal, augmenting an antidepressant with very low dose T4 or T3 often amplifies response.

Stimulants: Adding stimulants typically employed in the management of attention deficit disorder, such as Adderall (dextroamphetamine/amphetamine) or Ritalin (methylphenidate) can be effective in treating TRD. Before the first antidepressants were introduced to the United States market in the 1950s, stimulants were employed in the management of depression. Stimulants activate both the norepinephrine and dopamine systems.

Atypical Antipsychotics: A few of the second-generation antipsychotic medications, Zyprexa (olanzapine) and Abilify (aripiprazole) in particular, have shown effectiveness as augmenters to the traditional antidepressants. Abilify (aripiprazole) is FDA approved as an adjunct to antidepressants in the management of treatment-resistant unipolar depression.

Deplin (l-methylfolate): This is a folic acid type derivative that helps normalize amounts of neurotransmitters by aiding in their synthesis and subsequent generation. Depressed patients consistently have lower serum folate concentrations.

SAMe (S-adenosylmethionine): SAMe has certainly earned its stripes in recent years and is now considered by many to be one of the best natural alternatives in the treatment of mild to moderate depression. Well conducted studies have created quite a buzz, giving high marks to the effectiveness and tolerability of SAMe as an augmenting agent to traditional SSRIs and SNRIs. SAMe aids in methionine synthesis and acts as a precursor to neurotransmitter development—aiding in the improvement of nerve conduction. (More on SAMe in the Herbals and Supplements Chapter).

Omega-3 Fatty Acids: Fish oils are made up of EPA (eicosapentaenoic acid), critical in heart function, and DHA (docosahexaenoic acid), critical in brain function. These oils are found in fatty fish like salmon, mackerel, tuna and sardines and are available in supplements in gel cap form. Both DHA and EPA affect calcium, sodium, and potassium ion channels that regulate cellular electrical activity in the heart and the brain.

Omega-3 fatty acids have been well established with regard to improving nerve conduction, and they are well on their way to being recognized as effective in the management of depression by regulating neurotransmitters like serotonin and dopamine. Studies have shown a correlation between low levels of omega-3s and depression, and trials using omega-3s are showing promising results in the use of this supplement as a treatment for depression.

Symbyax (olanzapine/fluoxetine combination): Symbyax is a combination of the antipsychotic Zyprexa (olanzapine) and the antidepressant Prozac (fluoxetine). It is FDA approved for treatment-resistant depression. The olanzapine component of this drug is linked to weight gain, hyperglycemia, hyperlipidemia and hypercholesterolemia.

Combination Strategies

Antidepressants that can be used in combination with each other include: SSRIs + Wellbutrin; Remeron + Effexor; Remeron + SSRIs; Effexor + Wellbutrin; Effexor + SSRIs; Cymbalta + Wellbutrin.

What Else Influences a Less Than Adequate Response?

Monitor Dosage: Many depressed individuals just aren't dosed adequately. Sometimes a prescriber will need to adjust the dose to the FDA-approved maximum before results will be seen. If dosage maximums are reached and there is still little or no response, the next best step is to switch antidepressant classes. For example, if the individual has failed to respond to an SSRI, switch to an SNRI, an atypical like Wellbutrin (bupropion HCL) or even one of the hybrid antidepressants discussed in Chapter 6.

Monitor Compliance: Patients skip or forget doses of their medications particularly antidepressants, for a number of reasons, including the "stigma" associated with a diagnosis of depression as well as side effects and the cost of prescriptions.

Substance Abuse: Substance abuse complicates every aspect of the treatment of depression and interferes with the metabolism of antidepressants. As such, substance abusers with co-occurring depression have a decision to make: continue abusing illicit drugs and prescription medications with abuse potential or begin the process of abstaining. Period.

Undiagnosed Medical Disorders: Medical disorders such as diabetes, hypothyroidism, sleep apnea and restless legs syndrome can adversely affect antidepressant efficacy and therefore need to be thoroughly investigated.

Underlying Bipolar Disorder: Bipolar depression is a very tough nut to manage, and traditional antidepressants are all but considered failures in treating it. Additionally, antidepressants can cause manic switching and rapid cycling.

Unresolved Clinical Syndromes (Formerly Coded on Axis I): These may be related to the depressed individual only or to the family system in general. Also, the issue of "gain," primary or secondary, should be considered. The more intimate the relationship one has with their depression, the more difficult it will be to give up.

When pharmacological augmentation strategies don't work— either by adding drugs from a different class or combining them in typically effective pairs—other strategies need to be considered. These include "mechanical" strategies that warrant referrals to physicians or other skilled professionals knowledgeable in administering or performing these procedures. These strategies include:

Electroconvulsive Treatment (ECT): ECT came about as a procedure for treating depression when it was discovered that after a seizure patients often reported an improvement in mood and affect. In seizure disorder, neurotransmission is enhanced as a result of the repeated firing of neurons. ECT mimics a seizure, in this case an electrical therapeutic seizure lasting about 15 seconds.

ECT was in widespread use in the United States and England in the 1940s and 1950s, but experienced a decline from the 1950s to the 1970s with the advent of antidepressant medications. The procedure has been refined over the years and is performed under general anesthesia. It appears to carry no more risks than those of general anesthesia, and numerous reports confirm that ECT does not cause structural brain damage. The biggest single drawback to multiple treatments of ECT is memory loss, which can be either short-term or long- term. Still, ECT remains a somewhat controversial procedure due to sensationalism in movies and literature, and it is generally used only in those patients with severe depression who have not responded to antidepressants. ECT is an FDA-approved procedure.

Repetitive Transcranial Magnetic Stimulation (rTMS): This is an exciting tool in the research on brain function. Electrical activity in the brain is influenced by a pulsed magnetic field that is passed through a coil of wire encased in plastic and held close to the head. This magnetic field painlessly penetrates the scalp and skull, focusing on specific areas of the brain associated with mood disorders. The stimulation is made at regular intervals, thus the term "repetitive" TMS. Repetitive Transcranial Magnetic Stimulation likely stimulates underactive neurons and restores them to normal functioning. It is thought that the benefits of the TMS procedure are prolonged beyond the direct stimulation itself.

In studies, rTMS appears to change brain activity beyond the duration of the actual procedure. Also, the procedure differs from ECT in that it stimulates the brain in a focal manner, thereby preventing the grand mal seizure and minimizing the transitory memory loss associated with ECT.

In October, 2008 the FDA cleared the NeuroStar® TMS Therapy System by Neuronetics, Inc. for the treatment of depression. The standard course of FDA-approved treatment for the NeuroStar device is 36 treatments, performed daily for up to six weeks, and then tapered over a period of two to three weeks. A typical standard treatment is 40 minutes in duration from start to finish.

Vagal Nerve Stimulation (VNS): This mechanical strategy is an invasive procedure, initially used in epileptic patients and FDA-approved for TRD. VNS involves the implantation of a device called an NCP System in the upper chest. Electrodes are connected to the left cervical vagus nerve, through which electrical signals are delivered. This can facilitate neurotransmission, thus making this procedure potentially effective for the management of TRD.

Ketamine: Ketamine is a dissociative anesthetic with hallucinogenic properties. Its capacity to ameliorate depressive symptoms in people who have responded poorly to antidepressants has created quite a buzz in the psychiatry world. A study of 72 patients—presented at last year's annual meeting of the American Psychiatric Association—illustrated that more than half of the subjects reported fewer depressive symptoms after one intravenous dose of ketamine. This is a rather small sample size and other studies conducted have been similarly small. The "tale of the tape" when it comes to ketamine's effectiveness will be determined by the results of numerous controlled studies comparing ketamine with an active control. So, time will tell. Because of ketamine's rapid onset but short duration of action, it is conceivable that it could prove beneficial for severely depressed individuals who are acutely suicidal. Hallucinations are a side effect of ketamine, so this will have to be accounted for as ketamine-like products undergo development.

THE STARK REALITY OF MEDICATION TREATMENT RESISTANCE

Without a doubt, antidepressants have helped millions and millions of people emerge from the "pit" of depression—as one of my patients put it in a recent session together. Likewise, augmentation strategies have been a godsend to those who have reaped little or even no benefit whatsoever from monotherapy. But there's a potentially disconcerting downside to the use of medication in a round robin sort of fashion in search of the most appropriate combination. Here's an example:

> *"Joe, I'd like to ask you about the new antidepressant Fetzima. I've been taking it since January of this year, and although I got off to a good start with it, here I am beginning to taper off. My anxiety is as high as it's ever been, and I can barely stand being in my own skin. I have GAD and depression, and it now feels treatment-resistant. My anxiety is primarily the 'I dread everything type.' I have isolated myself mostly . . . I go to work, and come home. That's it. I see a psychiatric NP. Last month we tried Buspar in addition to Fetzima, but I had the worst heartburn and stopped taking it after a week. I have only had a good response to Effexor, however it stopped working in 2011. I have been in a downward spiral since then."*

I've received so many messages that read exactly the same way only the senders are different; and I believe that the number of antidepressants this person has tried exceeds what's mentioned in this missive.

Psychotropic medication resistance has doubled every five years since the early '80s and there has been a 3000 percent increase in reference literature that addresses treatment-resistant psychiatric circumstances, particularly with antidepressants, during this time frame. Affected people are increasingly being viewed as a complex series of neurobiological pathways that need to be untangled, activated, inhibited or massaged in some way. Given these resistance numbers, I'm hard- pressed to call this "evidence" of people being helped. I'm concerned that objectifying patients as mostly a compilation of the signs, symptoms and complaints they present with, slows progress toward getting them where they want or need to go. <u>Health is about helping patients achieve self-mastery, organizing their lives and taking charge of themselves, not reaching into the medication grab bag to find yet another drug to tame a pesky or emerging symptom.</u> Health is about promoting self-reliance and encouraging patients to explore what <u>they</u> need to do to get the engine of change moving steadily forward instead of subjecting them to the medication merry-go-round. Regardless of severity, every depressed individual with the intention of getting better needs to get moving and act. Circumstances of course will dictate the pace of progress.

Climbing the rungs on the neuroscience ladder yields a two-fold outcome. The science reaches new heights, providing us with bright, shiny, new medicinal therapies and strategies for using them, but also eventually encounters unforeseen roadblocks—testing the limits of how far it can take us. The paradox of evidence-based pharmacological practice is that far too many patients aren't getting better on medications, particularly antidepressants.

Ideally, various treatment disciplines would apply good, old-fashioned doses of common sense. Non-prescribers would caution patients about the limits of medications and focus on psychosocial interventions to generate improvement; and prescribers would exercise restraint and write prescriptions only when there is a <u>clear rationale</u> for medication use.

In his 1974 book *The Depressive Spectrum*, Dean Schuyler writes: "Most depressive episodes will run their course and terminate with virtually complete recovery without specific intervention." Still the case today, or old news?

CHAPTER 10

Other Treatment Paths for Managing Depression

Psychotherapy

Psychotherapy is the modality of choice for treating *reactive* depression and any of today's widely accepted models—traditional cognitive-behavioral; dialectical-behavioral; motivational interviewing; and mindfulness—are quite suitable choices. This of course is not primarily a psychotherapy book, so this section is not meant to be an exhaustive discussion of these widely accepted therapy models with outstanding track records of success. There are numerous seminars, workshops and training modules both live and online available to you to enhance your skills in these disciplines.

Work should begin from the position that the client is <u>not</u> damaged. Direct your efforts toward building on client strengths, instead of attempting to shore up weaknesses. Faulty thinking = ill feeling = faulty behavior = faulty outcomes is the scenario that has to change for the client to move productively forward.

Antidepressants don't work particularly well for reactive-type depressions because these drugs target biological deficits and therefore are unable to change the faulty belief systems that are characteristic of reactive depression. It's true that antidepressants may be able to alleviate some measure of the anxiety that accompanies stressful circumstances, but it's important to be clear: <u>Antidepressants are not **indicated** for psychosocial stress.</u> Those intent on using antidepressants to help ameliorate the distress associated with reactive, psychosocial-type events should think months of use—which is typically long enough for a stressful circumstance(s) to reach its conclusion. Medication <u>is</u> the mainstay of treatment for physical depression and all its influences with augmentation strategies a likely "must" due to physical compromise.

ADDRESS THE DEMONS OF DEPRESSION

I've identified four areas that are consistently problematic in the lives of depressed people. Helplessness, hopelessness, worthlessness, lack of motivation, pessimism and a life without pleasure—all core symptoms of depression—are fueled by these four demons. Depressed people have to be challenged to improve in these areas and should understand that they will need to push themselves and get moving pursuant to improvement. Motivation is an intrinsic decision that only they can make and execute.

Social Isolation

This is a circumstance that often flies under the radar not getting its just due and trumps all others when it comes to perpetuating depression. Isolation is the lead actor in the depression melodrama, ushering in the rest of the supporting cast (hopelessness, helplessness, etc.) and a glass- half-empty type of instance. It's generally not a planned thing; instead it morphs out of some of the accompanying physiological symptoms of depression, such as low energy, an absence of pleasurable activities in one's life and insomnia. Aloneness then summons negativity to join in, life becomes cocoon-like and few others—if any at all—are granted entry into the bubble.

Two of the biggest challenges confronting the treatment professional are: 1) finding effective ways to help the depressed client overcome inertia, and 2) encouraging the client to file for divorce from the thoughts perpetuating the doom and gloom, self-absorbed, "it's all about me" existence they're living. Keep in mind that both of these are counterintuitive to the ubiquitous notion among depressed clients that the depression itself keeps them from moving and that their circumstances are responsible for how they are feeling and behaving. Help these people by stressing the fact that isolating less means engaging more. This may sound obvious, but the rhythm of daily isolation has become so ingrained for some depressed people that they have tuned out developing a routine—which is precisely what they have to do.

Management is largely dependent on how immobilized the individual have become. Those with severe depression, who are not working or otherwise actively engaged, should of course take baby steps at first. This means poking a pin in their protective bubble and getting out of the house for something as simple as a walk to the curb or around the block to make a start. Adopting a routine beginning with a decision to be out of bed every day at a specific time, grooming, eating and then deciding on some structure for the balance of the day is the next part of the equation. Less is more at first to minimize discouragement while in a fragile state. So help them get started, then modify and adjust along the way. <u>Emphasize that they need living and breathing support to sustain them and that this can come from the obvious sources namely, family and friends, but also from conversations at the local coffee shop.</u> Talking to a trusted, caring family member or friend with established listening skills, together with psychotherapy, can go a long way to furthering the unburdening process.

Attitude

On the surface, attitude is the way we transmit our mood to others. When we are feeling optimistic, we convey a positive attitude, and for the most part, people usually respond favorably. When we are pessimistic, we send out negative vibes, and people tend to shun us. But attitude is more than the way we communicate our mood to others; it serves as the mind's eye—the way we see the world, so to speak. For example, a summer rain can be viewed as beautiful or ugly, a staff meeting as interesting or boring. Like using a camera, we take the snapshot of life we want to take.

Attitude never just stands still; it is an ongoing perceptual process requiring us to remain on constant guard. There is negativity all around us that can easily alter our perspective and affect our disposition. This makes it a challenge to keep positive thoughts within the inner circle of our thinking. Of course, no one is positive all of the time, and unbridled optimism—like that of the Pollyanna novels—is unrealistic and lacks genuineness. On the other hand, a chronically negative attitude dampens the spirit, saps energy, lessens enthusiasm, and compromises the immune system.

Poor attitude commonly accompanies depression, so some type of cognitive reframing is essential when working with depressed clients. Depressed people can experience the immobilizing inertia that I spoke about previously because of cynicism, pessimism and unrelenting negativity. They have to understand that to change the way they feel, they will have to adopt thinking and behavioral changes. Mindfulness techniques can be very helpful here. Focus on helping them set realistic expectations (they won't lose 20 pounds in one week), emphasize the benefits of taking on something new in their lives—big or small (learning that new language or how to play that musical instrument) and coach them to stop making comparisons by understanding that their own uniqueness counts for something potentially big-time. Another tip: suggest they read or listen to something funny every day. Newspaper comic strips and I Love Lucy episodes are classics.

Fear

Poor logic lies at the root of practically all fear, and the majority of what we experience as fear is a product of self-programming designed to make us feel helpless and run away. And when we identify with fear through our negative personal experiences, we are prone to examine the fear in an un-empowered way. Fear then becomes the worrier in our heads that interprets a situation to mean the worst will happen. This is all too common in depression, because depressed people tend to focus on the worst of possible outcomes for any given situation and will scan their environment to support these limiting beliefs.

Help clients to overcome this by encouraging them to first just notice the fear. Guide them to an understanding that when they feel afraid, they should take a step back and acknowledge it—without attempting to analyze, understand, assess or figure out the fear just yet. By doing so, they will give themselves some emotional space. Next, help them understand the difference between fear that is legitimately in the present from fear that is imagined. There's a big difference between actually losing one's job—and the financial concerns accompanying this—and believing one <u>will</u> lose their job. One is real; the other imagined. Then, do some probing by challenging the client with these questions: What is the fear really about? If the fear came true what would that mean? What is the fear preventing the client from doing?

An Imposter Mentality

Over the span of my many years of treating people with more manifestations of depression than I could shake a stick at, I've concluded that what is common about these depressions is this: Consistently, these folks feel inadequate most or all of the time, their self-worth is minimal at best, personal fulfillment is an abstract concept with which they are unfamiliar and they believe they're merely imposters masquerading through life awaiting the moment when they will be "found out," exposed and then humiliated. These phenomena drive their depression. This is not a "chemical imbalance" or "biological" problem, and medication is not the solution; it's a <u>faulty beliefs</u> problem. And it's worse today than ever before because the world is far more intricate and complex. We are literally overwhelmed with possible choices, everyone has a platform from which to sound off, and people we've modeled in numerous walks of life are being exposed as flimflams. <u>It comes down to this: Once anyone accepts the belief that they're unworthy or deficient, it is inevitable that they will eventually perceive themselves as a failure, decompensate and move toward some manifestation of depression, anxiety or other form of escapism.</u>

So why does this happen? How do people get themselves in this position? For two reasons:

1. **Playing the same old tapes over and over.** Some people are not able to get past the upbraiding, rebuking, chastising and berating unleashed on them by significant others throughout their lives—often beginning in early childhood. The constancy of harshness and criticism shapes belief systems that serve as springboards launching them into an all-out assault on themselves. And even though they may be very different people now, these admonition tapes continue to play in their heads at off-the-chart decibel levels.

2. **Finding the dislike or disapproval of others uncomfortable and hard to accept.** Many, many people think that their worthiness is contingent upon having to continually prove themselves to themselves and others. But when situations arise where they believe they are a disappointment, they tune in the negative at the expense of the positive. That is, in spite of overwhelmingly positive outcomes, they hear one bad thing about them or get one negative evaluation, and the floodgates of negativity are unleashed: "See, I told you so!" "Why did I risk putting myself out there?" "Why did I think anyone would listen to me in the first place?" "When someone really good at this appears, I'll be a goner!" The takeaway: Beliefs always guide behaviors.

So what to do about such self-worth and image busters? Here are seven key recommendations for your clients or for anyone—including yourself—experiencing depression, dysphoria or anxiety as a result of low self-worth or lagging personal fulfillment:

> **Organize and Prioritize.** The very first step is realizing that personal esteem and feeling fulfilled is all about control of your own life. And this control is contingent upon your ability to organize your life. This means being able to access what you need when you need it and being in a position to concentrate on your most important priorities.
>
> Once you're organized, your personal control grows—this in turn, enhances your personal power (flexibility, versatility, influence, and so on); more power leads to more success—which enriches your self-esteem. So, get organized mentally and physically,

and cease telling yourself and others that you're "overwhelmed," or have "writer's block," or feel "lost." All of this is negative nonsense and self-defeating. By organizing your life and thereby gaining the control you desire, you'll free yourself from the "doom and gloom loop" and launch yourself into the "success loop."

The first step toward getting organized is to have immediate and unencumbered accessibility to what you need to get through your day successfully. Some people claim they know where everything is in their messy house or office, but eventually this becomes self-defeating because thriving in such an environment will become ever more challenging. Acting promptly and efficiently requires order, otherwise chaos will eventually rule. And chaos is distracting and makes for a bad impression particularly to clients, leaving the impression that if you can't order your own life, how could you possibly help order theirs or assist them with their concerns.

Another important step is eliminating time thieves. The headliner here is so often the "to do" list. Those devoted to such lists record what needs to be done today, tomorrow, the day after, next week, ad infinitum - an endlessly growing protoplasm of sorts that never stops reproducing. When everything on the list is perceived as a priority, then of course, nothing winds up being a priority; and the mere length of the list is so intimidating that it invites inertia. Worse, listing things becomes an end in and of itself, creating the false impression that <u>some kind of action has been taken.</u>

Give the "to do" list a break, here's how:

1. Record anything you believe you must do, personal or professional, into a <u>physical</u> calendar of some sort. Assign a date and time for completion and treat it as sacrosanct, that is, outside of some acute emergency, it will get done.

2. Set a maximum of five or six tasks as a daily limit and tweak completion of these to match your life style. Determine when you're at your "output best" and work hardest then. Morning? Afternoon? Early evening?

3. Don't set your sights on completing any one task in a singular time frame. Mix and shift task completion to stave off boredom and distraction by "chunking" them down. You'll feel less

overwhelmed when writing a lengthy report if you write in 30 minute segments. If you're seeking referral business and have 20 prospects, call four of them per day over a five-day span.

It's accurate to say that making lists and crossing out completed items provides a sense of accomplishment, but if you are intent on increasing your efficiency, lists will inevitably bog you down and hang around your neck like an albatross.

Monitor self-talk. Write down this statement, post it in an easily recognizable place and recite it out loud 3–5 times per day: "I have tremendous value which can help people personally and professionally, and I'd be remiss not to approach as many people as I can with this opportunity." A statement like this affirms the belief that you <u>already</u> possess value from which others may benefit. There is no question that you believe you are valid when using this "I" message. The belief though is no more than a self-affirmation unless you take this action step—approaching as many people as possible such that they don't miss out on all the good stuff in store for them by associating with you.

Strive for success, not perfection. Every product we produce, service we offer or project we develop is subject to becoming flawed once we expose it to outside forces—unless you want to keep it completely to yourself. Subjecting anything we believe worthwhile to revision after revision, rewrite after rewrite and meeting upon meeting before unleashing it to those who could benefit from it is just a shame. Why? Because with no imposed limits on these perfection steps, it will never reach the hands of those eagerly awaiting it. Tweaking something over and over rarely makes it better—only different from the last change. So concentrate on just getting it out there, assess what happens and <u>then makes changes accordingly</u>. Believe me, perfectionism will wear you down and wear you out because you'll never get there.

Stop saying "Yes" when you really mean "No." Taking on and fighting every battle that comes your way all but ensures that you will lose most of them. Allowing yourself to be coerced into thinking and acting someone else's way are surefire steps to diminish what's important to <u>you</u>. If someone is seemingly out to damage your reputation or is attacking your value system, fight back in every reasonable legal and ethical way to get it stopped. But ignore the nitpickers and those with a bent toward spouting off on anything—particularly if unsolicited. To be at your best to deliver value to those that mean the most demands <u>putting yourself first.</u> This is humility well-placed. It reserves you for those to whom you want to say "Yes" and frees you from those who want you to say "Yes." Slings and arrows come from all directions and there is no shortage of those with designs on you to enrich themselves, placing them in a better position. Saying "No" isn't self-serving; it is self-liberating because it helps order and align your priorities.

Understand and display confidence. The essence of confidence starts with believing in yourself for sure, but it also means having unwavering faith in your ability to help others benefit from your value in areas where you feel fully qualified. We're not born with confidence, instead it's a trait that is cultivated and shaped through our beliefs and experiences beginning in early childhood. Confidence is gained through positive, reinforcing feedback from significant others, friends and peers close to us regarding the value of our beliefs, self-worth and abilities. It can be self-earned through our own attempts to master something through repeated efforts often resulting in failure at first, followed by starting anew, modifications or fine tuning before eventually achieving the success we're seeking. Initial success then begets more of the same and we're off and running at full throttle and hitting on all cylinders. You know you're confident when you completely believe in your ability to help others and then demonstrate that ability by objectively improving their position. Once attained, confidence <u>must</u> be displayed and doing so is not a sign of arrogance or an absence of humility. Confident people lead, not follow, and aren't discouraged by criticisms and challenges from others. And they fully comprehend this: they must blow their own horn so that others will hear their music.

Know your value. Believe it. There is something special about you, and your uniqueness counts for something potentially big time. Do you know what it is? If you do, are you connecting with and demonstrating this value to those who can benefit from it? Don't permit yourself to remain a best kept secret.

Nobody wins, certainly not you nor those whose positions would be markedly improved by working with you. If you really don't know your value, start with this exercise: Make a list of five things you consider yourself either good or great at. No self-censoring when composing this list. After listing these, take a moment to reflect on how it feels to actually see your attributes, assets, skills and accomplishments staring back at you. Then take this list and exploit it to its fullest possible potential. Personal fulfillment is at its most powerful when you set your sights on accomplishing or achieving something and then going about the business of doing it. Self-worth soars, confidence mounts and success begets more of the same. And when these factors coalesce, you'll no longer feel like an imposter waiting to be cast aside when the winners show up. You're now one of these winners—no longer a stand-in for those in the starring roles.

Don't sell yourself short. Believing that you're short on substance and long on inferiority has few peers when it comes to feeding the imposter mentality. Really, why convince yourself that your contributions are inferior? Most of those who have accomplished much haven't wowed us with something "Einsteinish." Instead, they staked their claim for their positions and beliefs and then set out to demonstrate why they work and who can benefit from them. Different slants on existing ideas and concepts have molded many people into thought leaders. And these people often do this by being controversial and contrarian where appropriate—making them stand out from the sea of sameness. You can do the same. Develop it, support its rationale, take it out for a test drive, assess the results and then launch, modify or scrap as you see fit. Keep going. And it is okay if some people are ticked off with you and don't like your ideas. This is often when you're striking the right chord.

Diet

You have likely heard the phrase "you are what you eat." Now since life is indisputably multi-dimensional, the "you are" part of this phrase is obviously restricted as there are many other contenders that shape you. How and what you eat though is way atop the hit parade. No one lives a prosperous life without good health, because health is the bedrock, the foundation that propels you forward (or not). Bellies are getting bigger and bigger in this country, and yes, in some instances obesity is unavoidable, but for most of us it is. I could wax ineloquent in dietician-like terms about food and beverage consumption but won't because you've heard such refrains ad nauseam. You know what you should eat and drink more of and less of. Temptations, hooks and siren calls abound when it comes to food and beverage.

Today's typical American diet which is high in processed foods is nearly devoid of essential elements like magnesium and zinc, not to mention many others. Foods high in the "bad fat" category encourage not only weight gain but also a sedentary lifestyle which can lead to increasing lethargy and listlessness. Excessive sugar intake causes fluctuations in blood sugar levels, increasing the risk of developing type 2 diabetes. All of these factors are deleterious to mood in the long run. People with depression should be encouraged to take healthy eating recommendations seriously and even consult a dietician or nutritionist. With such professional guidance, changes to a healthier and balanced eating regimen is not only doable, but it can be accomplished without undue sacrifice.

Exercise

While on the subject of good health as the bedrock and foundation of prosperity, need I extol the virtues of moving your body? Every day is better when a cardiovascular component is part of your daily living. What's not to like about being fit and better oxygenated. Mental acuity benefits abound as well. You'll find travel easier and have greater endurance, fewer bouts of illness, and more sustained energy day in and day out. As with healthy eating, mood benefits abound. Exercise promotes endorphin release and getting in shape instills a sense of accomplishment. Group exercise curbs social isolation, encourages relationship development and promotes an attitude of "we're all getting fit together."

Severely depressed people should take baby steps at first, beginning first with a walk outside, then around the block and so on, improving their tolerance levels along the way. We all have to move.

God, Religion, Spirituality

A study published in the American Journal of Psychiatry examined the effect of religion and spirituality on depression. Those participating in the study who claimed that religion was important to them had only one-tenth the risk of experiencing depression compared to those not holding religion in high esteem. And whether you believe in evolution or intelligent design, people throughout the annals of history have commented that religious affiliation or living with an active spiritual component is centering, grounding, helps order their lives, and fosters moral discipline and restraint. And with a belief system firmly rooted in the concept that God is good, structured church affiliation serves as a safe haven where grace, strength and guidance to face the tribulations and challenges of life can be sought, while offering thanks to a supreme being. The dividends of worship then, are peace and contentment.

There are numerous resources available—ranging from models of integrating faith and psychology, to how to work clinically with various modalities. You can find cognitive-behavioral practitioners and learn how they integrate religion and spirituality into practice as well as those employing psychoanalytic or family systems methodologies. Even the American Psychiatric Association is publishing information about spirituality and religiousness. The key is figuring out how to utilize these without being imposing or even worse, insolent.

Bright Light

Lack of sunlight has been linked with mood disorders—especially Seasonal Affective Disorder (SAD). Seasonal Affective Disorder appears to be caused by our bodies' response to seasonal changes. It seems our daily circadian rhythms shift with the seasons, partly in response to changes in patterns of sunlight. When the daylight hours shorten during late fall and winter, some individuals experience a biochemical imbalance in the brain. From a treatment perspective, light therapy—also known as phototherapy—has proven to be effective in up to 35 percent of diagnosed cases. With light therapy, the patient is exposed to a very bright light—at least 10 times the intensity of ordinary domestic lighting—for up to four hours a day (though one to two hours is the average).

The patient typically sits two to three feet away from a specially designed light box. Reputable light-box manufacturers include Bio-Light, Sun-Box and Northern Light Technologies. This bright light activates the circuits in the brain that cause mood-boosting chemical reactions. While sitting in front of the light box, the patient can engage in normal activities, such as reading and eating. Treatment is usually effective within three or four days, and the benefits continue with daily use. Even for those living without seasonal issues, venturing out and getting a healthy dose of sunshine each day can produce a brightening effect on mood. And it discourages social isolation. So let there be light in your life—it's a free mood booster!

JOE'S 7-POINT PLAN FOR TREATING DEPRESSION

1. **Get depressed clients thinking and behaving in such a way that they are better able to thrive.** Encourage them to stop talking "overwhelm," "the world's out to get them" or "it's somebody else's fault." That's all negative nonsense which serves as a vehicle for self-sabotage, keeping

them in the "doom loop." Get them in the "success loop" by encouraging them to socially isolate less, improve their attitude and better understand the unrealistic aspects of their fears. All of these demons fuel helplessness, hopelessness and worthlessness.

2. **The bulk of your work should focus on helping the client "strengthen their strengths" not shore up their weaknesses.** Most clients will light up when I ask about their strengths and how these have helped them get as far as they have in life. On the other hand, inquiring about their weaknesses and suggesting a plan for improving them invites a sense of dread. It's much more effective and efficient to have the client identify and utilize tools for beating their depression that are already in their skill set than to have them start from scratch to improve in areas in which they are unaccomplished and disinterested. Don't introduce resistance into treatment; invite cooperation.

3. **Get depressed clients moving and doing things. Depression attracts rumination and inertia like a magnet.** Getting them moving and doing something—anything productive, interesting or fun—Serves a viable distraction. Inactivity feeds malaise which in turn feeds dysphoria; activity keeps it at bay and out of mind.

4. **If the depression is severe, treat with medication.** Once a depressed individual begins exhibiting physiological symptom changes such as a change in appetite or sleep, energy loss, cognitive fog or demonstrable melancholia, medication intervention becomes a mainstay. Debilitation invites resistance to behavioral interventions and cognitive-based psychotherapy, so medication is warranted to get the client into a better position physically.

5. **Assuming some measure of improvement via medication, get the client moving and doing things.** Discourage an attitude of using medication as an end-all. It's not and you need to be assertive about this. Medication does not change behavior; it can, however, light the path to improvement.

6. **Reevaluate the need for medication going forward.** It's common for a depressed client to not respond to the first regimen tried because there is no one drug, combination, algorithm or augmentation strategy that applies to all. Trial and error, mixing and matching rule.

7. **Guide them toward being accountable for healthy eating, regular exercise and the benefits of incorporating God, spirituality and religion into their everyday living.**

CHAPTER 11

Mood-Stabilizing Agents

Lithium was the first mood-stabilizing medication approved by the FDA for the treatment of acute mania and hypomania. It might well be the "gold standard" in the treatment of mania, as well as for the maintenance treatment of bipolar I and II. Although lithium has its drawbacks, it is considered a first-line agent. It is generally safe and effective when carefully monitored and its side effects appropriately managed. Two other medication classes with mood-stabilizing properties used to treat bipolar disorders are the anticonvulsants a nd the atypical antipsychotics. These medications are often used in combination with psychotherapy for a significant and positive impact on this biologically based illness.

LITHIUM

The mood-stabilizing properties of lithium were first noted in the 1800s, when physicians used it for not only treating anxiety, but also gout and seizures. In 1949, an Australian psychiatrist, John Cade, published the first paper on lithium's usefulness for treating acute mania. In his experiments, Cade had earlier observed that lithium had a calming effect on guinea pigs. He then tried it on human subjects and found their mania subsided within a week. It took a while, however, for lithium to gain acceptance in American medicine; government approval did not come until 1970. Then increased marketing of the drug quickly followed under the brand names Eskalith and Lithobid.

Today, more than 50 years later, lithium's workings are still unclear. One theory is that lithium normalizes mania initially through its effects on norepinephrine. When fight or flight is activated, synaptic levels of norepinephrine tend to increase. According to this theory, lithium acts as a fight-or-flight deactivator by increasing norepinephrine reuptake. Lithium's effect on serotonin is theorized to be responsible for its role in managing depressive episodes of bipolar disorder. Because some bipolar patients demonstrate low concentrations of serotonin, lithium may contribute to enhancing the actions of serotonin by increasing levels of tryptophan, a building block of serotonin. Lithium has well documented efficacy in preventing relapse in bipolar disorder. Lithium reduces the risk of suicide and suicide attempts associated with bipolar disorder, though it does not reduce the risk found in the general population. This is important, because about 1 percent of those with bipolar disorder attempt suicide each year.

One drawback to lithium is its slow onset of action: It typically requires 5 to 14 days, with full stabilization taking up to several months. Another drawback is lithium's narrow therapeutic index, meaning the therapeutic dose is very close to the toxic dose. Most patients must reach a level between 1.0 and 1.2 milliequivalents per liter (mEq/L) to see results. However, the toxic level can begin around 1.5 mEq, even lower. For this reason, lithium requires careful blood-level monitoring.

Generally speaking, the starting dose of lithium is 600 mg to 900 mg daily, administered in divided doses. During acute manic states, daily doses can range from 1200 mg to 2400 mg, with most patients requiring 600 mg to 1800 mg daily after stabilization. It is recommended that blood-level monitoring be done once every 7 days for the first few weeks, then once every 3 months after stabilization. Laboratory tests to check thyroid and kidney function are warranted before lithium treatment begins. Lithium use can lead to a decrease in thyroid production, so it may be useful to obtain a yearly thyroid-stimulating hormone (TSH) level to check for this. Symptoms of hypothyroidism include weight gain, fatigue, dry skin and intolerance to cold. It is generally not necessary to stop the lithium, since providing additional thyroid hormone in a daily oral preparation can easily manage decreased thyroid function.

Baseline kidney-function testing is also recommended prior to the initiation of lithium use. Lithium bypasses liver metabolism and depends solely on the kidney for excretion from the body. In the absence of healthy kidney functioning, lithium levels can rise rapidly, and toxicity then becomes a major issue. Though there is concern regarding lithium use and kidney damage, such damage is for the most part rare.

Recommended laboratory tests include:

- Na (Sodium)
- Ca (Calcium)
- P (Phosphorous)

- EKG
- Creatinine
- Urinalysis
- Complete Blood Count
- Thyroid Function

Possible Side Effects

Lithium's side effects range from those that are relatively benign and temporary to more serious ones that can lead to toxicity, coma, and even death.

Side Effects of Lithium	
Most Common:	**Most Severe:**
Diabetes insipidus	Hypothyroidism
Excessive urination	Kidney dysfunction
Weight gain	Confusion
Nausea, vomiting, diarrhea	Coma
Aggravation of acne	

Common side effects include nausea, diarrhea, vomiting, thirst, excessive urination, weight gain and fine hand tremor. A benign, reversible increase in white blood cell count frequently occurs with lithium use. This ordinarily does not rise to clinical significance nor does it require lithium discontinuation. Chronic use side effects include hypothyroidism, goiter, and rarely, kidney damage. And signs of toxicity include lethargy, ataxia, slurred speech, shock, delirium, coma and death.

Lithium elimination from the body is affected by excessive sodium loss. Sodium loss through dehydration, diarrhea, increased perspiration or diuretic medication use can trigger lithium retention in the body that could reach toxic levels. Accordingly, baseline kidney function tests are warranted, and regular monitoring is imperative.

ANTICONVULSANTS

Another class of mood stabilizers used to manage bipolar disorder is the anticonvulsants, utilized for more than 35 years in the management of seizure disorder. Similar to lithium, the exact functioning of how anticonvulsants treat bipolar disorder remains unclear. The chief suspect, however, is the anticonvulsants' ability to enhance the actions of GABA, the primary inhibitory neurotransmitter in the central nervous system (as previously discussed).

Several anticonvulsants have demonstrated efficacy and are widely prescribed. These include Depakote (divalproex), Lamictal (lamotrigine), Tegretol (carbamazepine) and Topamax (topiramate).

Depakote (divalproex) is considered—like lithium—a first-line agent for mania and is the likely agent of choice for rapid cycling. Several studies have indicated that it works more quickly than lithium and may be better tolerated. Depakote (divalproex) is also excellent for treating rage reactions and extreme mood instability in bipolar disorder and disruptive behaviors associated with conduct disorder, borderline personality disorder, autism and attention deficit hyperactivity disorder. The drug is typically ineffective in the treatment of bipolar depression.

The main side effects of Depakote (divalproex) include sedation, dizziness, drowsiness, blurred vision and coordination problems. Gastrointestinal side effects include nausea, vomiting, diarrhea, and abdominal pain. Taking the medication with food or milk may lessen these side effects. Depakote (divalproex) can also cause interference with blood clotting; liver toxicity in children (although this is primarily associated with those taking multiple psychiatric medications); weight gain in approximately 50 percent of patients seems to be dose-related; and pancreatitis, with its primary symptom of abdominal pain. Any reports of abdominal pain should be immediately referred to a physician. Another possible side effect of Depakote (divalproex) is polycystic ovarian syndrome (PCOS) in women of childbearing age, which can lead to decreased fertility, weight gain, menstrual irregularities and endocrine problems such as excessive hair growth.

Lamictal (lamotrigine) is approved for acute and maintenance treatment of bipolar illness and for the management of rapid cycling bipolar disorder. Lamictal (lamotrigine) is purportedly less effective for mania and more effective for the depressive phase of a mood swing. There is growing concern that this drug is not as effective for acute bipolar depression as previously thought, and that its efficacy is better suited to reducing the risk of future bipolar depressive episodes.

Central nervous system side effects of Lamictal (lamotrigine) include sedation, dizziness, drowsiness, blurred vision and coordination problems. Gastrointestinal side effects include nausea, vomiting, diarrhea and abdominal pain. A potentially serious side effect of Lamictal (lamotrigine) is rash development, including Stevens-Johnson syndrome. This does not necessarily mean that all rashes associated with Lamictal (lamotrigine) use are linked to Stevens-Johnson, but it is something that should be monitored. With Stevens-Johnson, tissue undergoes necrolysis and takes on the appearance of a third or fourth degree burn. Rash development, which occurs in about 10 percent of patients, seems to be related to how fast this medication is started and subsequently titrated upward. Current clinical guidelines recommend that Lamictal (lamotrigine) doses be gradually increased to typical daily maximums of 100 mg to 200 mg over a six-week period. If any manifestation of a rash appears, this drug should be discontinued immediately and a physician consulted.

Tegretol (carbamazepine) is effective for mania but is generally considered a second-line agent to Depakote (divalproex). Like Depakote (divalproex), Tegretol (carbamazepine) is unproven in the treatment of bipolar depression. For years it has been a very effective anticonvulsant for use in the management of grand mal seizures. It is still used on occasion to manage aggressive outbursts in children. Central nervous system side effects include sedation, dizziness, drowsiness, blurred vision and coordination problems. Gastrointestinal side effects include nausea, vomiting, diarrhea and abdominal pain.

Tegretol (carbamazepine) is also linked to the potentially serious side effect of agranulocytosis, causing a decrease in white blood cell count that can lead to the development of opportunistic infection.

Topamax (topiramate) lacks efficacy in well-controlled studies in the management of bipolar disorder; in effect it has basically failed as a mood stabilizer, unlike the other drugs mentioned above. Weight loss is a side effect of Topamax (topiramate), so it is used on occasion to help with weight gain caused by other psychotropics. Also, because of its effects on calcium channel signaling and GABA, it is used in the treatment of migraine headaches and has received FDA approval for this. Topamax (topiramate) has also demonstrated some short-term efficacy in alcohol dependence by reducing alcohol cravings after the withdrawal phase.

A potentially significant side effect of Topamax (topiramate) involves cognitive difficulties—cognitive "fog"—as well as memory disturbance and word-finding difficulties. Rare cases of glaucoma and kidney stones have also surfaced.

Topamax (topiramate) Cognitive difficulties—mental "fog"—as well as memory disturbance and word-finding difficulties. Rare cases of glaucoma and kidney stones have also surfaced.

Side Effects of Anticonvulsants	
Drug	**Side Effects**
Tegretol (carbamazepine)	Sedation, dizziness, drowsiness, blurred vision and coordination problems. Nausea, vomiting, diarrhea and abdominal pain. Linked to potentially serious side effect of agranulocytosis, causing significant decrease in white blood cell count, which can lead to opportunistic infections.
Depakote (divalproex)	Sedation, dizziness, drowsiness, blurred vision and coordination problems. Nausea, vomiting, diarrhea and abdominal pain. Interference with blood clotting; weight gain in approximately 50 percent of patients; pancreatitis; possible liver toxicity in children; polycystic ovarian syndrome (PCOS) in women of childbearing age.
Lamictal (lamotrigine)	Sedation, dizziness, drowsiness, blurred vision and coordination problems. Nausea, vomiting, diarrhea, and abdominal pain. Rash development, including Stevens-Johnson syndrome (potentially serious).
Topamax (topiramate)	Cognitive difficulties—mental "fog"—as well as memory disturbance and word-finding difficulties. Rare cases of glaucoma and kidney stones have also surfaced.

Other Anticonvulsants

Currently, other anticonvulsants are considered alternative or augmenting agents for bipolar disorder. On the whole, these anticonvulsants lack well-controlled clinical studies supporting their first-line or, in some cases, second-line use in bipolar disorder. These include Neurontin (gabapentin), Gabitril (tiagabine), Trileptal (oxcarbazepine), Felbatol (felbamate), Keppra (levetiracetam) and Lyrica (pregabalin).

ATYPICAL ANTIPSYCHOTICS

Newer, atypical antipsychotics are gaining increasingly widespread acceptance in the management of bipolar disorder. Zyprexa (olanzapine) and Abilify (aripiprazole) are both FDA-approved for acute and maintenance treatment of bipolar mania. Another atypical antipsychotic, Symbyax (olanzapine and fluoxetine), is FDA-approved for the treatment of depressive episodes associated with bipolar disorder. All of the atypical antipsychotics currently available in the United States—with the notable exception of Clozaril (clozapine)—are FDA-approved for acute bipolar mania. FDA approvals are routinely under review and are subject to change, so it is wise to consult product literature and even the FDA website for the most accurate and up-to-date information.

The pharmacological treatment of bipolar disorder is to say the least, all over the place, and clinician disagreement as to which medication should be utilized in what particular instance is vast. So to allay some of this confusion, what follows is a summary of the most recent advances in medicating bipolar disorder:

- Lithium is <u>clearly</u> the most efficacious **single agent** for managing bipolar mania.
- Combining lithium with Depakote (divalproex) does increase efficacy—although not markedly.
- The lithium/Depakote (divalproex) combination therefore is optimal in bipolar mania.
- Although FDA approved, second-generation antipsychotics are not yet considered first line treatment for mania.
- Seroquel (quetiapine), Seroquel XR (quetiapine XR), Latuda (lurasidone) (although very expensive) and the Prozac/Zyprexa combination Symbyax, stand out for bipolar depression. Make no mistake, bipolar depression is tough to treat effectively—much tougher than manic episodes. Don't underestimate lithium's effectiveness in bipolar depression.
- Traditional antidepressants have practically nothing to offer for bipolar depression. They don't necessarily cause a switch to mania but can induce hyperexcitability which masquerades as mania-like.

TREATMENT-RESISTANT BIPOLAR DISORDER: A FORMIDABLE FOE

Treatment resistance in bipolar disorder is very common. Even with optimal care, which includes medication combinations, 50 percent of bipolar individuals who achieve symptom remission will relapse within two years. And although clinically familiar, the concept of treatment resistance lacks a standard definition upon which clinicians and diagnosticians can reliably agree. Another area of disagreement is pharmacological management. Combining medications is a routine practice and the number of potential combinations is considerable. There is little sound clinical evidence to drive decisions about which medications to use first, and how these should be dosed. In short, both the notion and management of treatment-resistant bipolar disorder depends upon whom you ask and their successes and failures with treating it.

Headwinds

When working with these patients, you are likely to encounter some or even most of the following: suicide risk is highest among all psychiatric disorders at 20 percent; 25 percent have an alcohol problem. Most will find their way to your offices by way of the criminal justice system or because they've taken unreasonable risks and are considered a danger to themselves or others, particularly during the manic phase.

These patients typically don't present to treatment during the manic phase because mania is a desired state. If they do, ego concerns, arrogance, a sense of entitlement, a lack of awareness, and an inability to calculate the consequences of their behavior often accompany the classic manic symptoms. Confirming a diagnosis could literally take years because these patients don't tend to volunteer information, are poor historians and need constant redirection. Clinicians who are intolerant of unruly behavior can be worn down quickly by these presentations. Clear boundaries should be established from the outset of treatment.

Treatment-resistant Bipolar Mania

Historically, lithium and certain anticonvulsants have been employed as first-line agents for acute mania with antipsychotics reserved for more resistant, very ill, psychotic patients. However, the spectrum of FDA-sanctioned uses for the second-generation antipsychotics in bipolar disorder continues to expand—with some prescribers now utilizing them for moderately ill manic individuals. For truly resistant conditions, Clozaril (clozapine) and ECT are recommended. Despite the innumerable mix-and-match medication strategies for treatment- resistant mania—many of which demonstrate little if any efficacy in comparative studies—the Lithium/Depakote (divalproex) combination still remains optimal in mania prevention.

Treatment-resistant Bipolar Depression

There are few treatments that have demonstrated efficacy in bipolar depression and it is proving to be a tough nut to treat successfully. Only two medications, Seroquel (quetiapine) and Symbyax (a Prozac/Zyprexa combination) have been approved. Other recommended agents are lithium and Lamictal (lamotrigine).

Traditional antidepressants have little if any benefit in bipolar depression and may be associated with a switch to mania. In particular, the serotonin and norepinephrine (SNRI) agents are associated with an even higher risk of switching. The SNRIs include Effexor (venlafaxine), Cymbalta (duloxetine) and Pristiq (desvenlafaxine). For patients who do not respond to the drugs of choice listed above, prescriber creativity in finding a combination that can help becomes a must. Lithium, Seroquel (quetiapine) and Lamictal (lamotrigine) can be used in combination with one another. Also, Vagus Nerve Stimulation (VNS)—discussed in Chapter 9—has demonstrated efficacy.

OTHER REMEDIES

Medication should always be combined with intensive cognitive- behavioral psychotherapies that include supportive family members whenever possible. Psychotherapy should appeal to patients' "better angels" and help them harness their creativity by channeling it toward more productive outcomes. Neurofeedback (NFB), a technique by which subjects learn to self-regulate their own neural activity through the use of brain activity displays in real-time, has been associated with positive outcomes.

Treatment-resistant bipolar disorder is highly nuanced, complex, and most certainly does not lend itself to black-or-white judgments when it comes to medication management. Polypharmacy will likely be necessary since complications and co-morbidities such as substance abuse are the rule rather than the exception. The most important consideration when employing multiple drug agents is to conceptualize a reason for each medication choice. And clinicians must stress medication compliance as a means to quality of life and survival.

PSYCHOTHERAPY FOR BIPOLAR DISORDER

It is all but impossible to conduct results-oriented psychotherapy with a bipolar patient whose medication management is inadequate. Manic symptoms breed poor insight and judgment, and the inability to accommodate and assimilate even the most basic tenets of psychotherapy in a meaningful way. Combine these factors with the DIGFAST symptoms that define the manic spectrum and there's virtually nothing to be gained.

Bipolarity comes with significant challenges for the clinician employing psychotherapy. First, the psychotherapist has to treat two very different mood states—mania and depression. Second, mania is often a desired condition that a patient wants to continue experiencing rather than not, and the desire to remain manic often results in missed appointments and unaccountability. Also, the low energy and excessive sleeping symptoms of bipolar depression can exacerbate social isolation and poor attitude. Compounding all this is that the patient can "switch" at any time biologically or the switch may be induced by substance abuse of some sort. The three components of a psychotherapy model that potentially can make a positive difference for the affected patient are:

1. **Cognitive-behavioral therapy** which concentrates on helping the patient understand the ramifications of distorted thinking and irrational activity; emphasizes the likely lifetime prevalence of bipolar disorder and the importance of accepting this along with long-term medication compliance; and learning new ways to cope with the disorder.

2. **Family-centered therapy** which focuses on the family's ability to increasingly cope more effectively with the identified patient family member and recognize the warning signs of symptom worsening in their loved one; and developing communication and problem-solving skills within the family structure.

3. **Rhythm therapy** which teaches the patient how to better stabilize and organize daily routines and adhere to eating, exercise and sleep/wake schedules.

What You and Your Clients Need To Know

The manic phase of bipolar disorder carries a peculiar treatment challenge that most other mental disorders do not: Because mania is a desirable and enjoyable state for many, if not most patients, medication noncompliance is a particular hazard during these episodes. Repeatedly starting and discontinuing mood stabilizers results in erratic blood levels of these medications and a subsequent decrease in their effectiveness. This, in turn, can lead to an increased susceptibility for the occurrence of future episodes, a progressive worsening of symptoms, and a heightened mortality risk. Therefore, clinicians must stress compliance and taking medication as prescribed as a means to quality of life and survival.

CASE STUDY: "A VERY IMPORTANT MAN"

Steven is a 25-year-old flooring and carpet sales representative referred to you by his primary care physician. He called your office a day earlier seeking an immediate appointment to discuss his recent bouts of stress, anxiety and sleeplessness. When Steven arrives at your office, he is abrupt, abrasive, and demanding. He tells the administrative assistant that he is a "very important man" who expects to be seen by you "right now." The assistant notifies you of his arrival, but not before he attempts to pass around carpet samples to other clients in the waiting room.

Steven is unshaven, possesses a detectable body odor, and his clothing is wrinkled. He reports that his father has been "in and out of the nut house" as long as he can remember and that one of his older brothers is an alcoholic. Steven reveals no other psychiatric history. He is, by self-report, single, never married and without children. He has recently been promoted to senior sales representative at the flooring company owned by his oldest brother.

During the interview, Steven rises from his chair on several occasions and paces incessantly in front of your office window. He states that his recent anxiety and insomnia is entirely his brother's fault. Steven desires to take the family carpet company "global," he continues, but his brother has rejected this plan because, "he thinks too small." Steven's speech is pressured, and his thought processes are disorganized and accompanied by a flight of ideas. Considering that Steven's symptoms may be indicative of a manic episode, you refer him to one of the psychiatrists in your agency for additional evaluation.

Diagnostic Considerations

The psychiatrist conducts his own independent assessment and concludes that the inappropriate behavior Steven displayed in the patient waiting area, as well as the overall symptom intensity, warrants medication management. The physician explains to Steven that he has a condition that is well known for the symptoms and behavior he has been experiencing. The psychiatrist suggests a trial of lithium beginning with 300 mg twice daily to be taken at mealtimes. The psychiatrist stressed the importance of monitoring Steven's lithium levels every 3 to 7 days for the first several weeks of treatment, and that the maintenance level to be achieved is 1.0 to 1.2mEq/l.

TREATMENT COURSE

Over the next six weeks, Steven's lithium dose is increased to 1800 mg daily. Steven responds favorably to lithium treatment, and the doctor suggests he should remain on long-term maintenance management, possibly indefinitely. Throughout the treatment process, Steven's psychiatrist secures all of the appropriate informed consents and engages Steven in a detailed discussion of the possible side effects of lithium use. The physician also emphasizes that for as long as Steven remains in treatment, he will need occasional lithium blood-level monitoring, thyroid function tests, and kidney-function tests, probably about once every 3 months.

Dosage Range Chart—Mood Stabilizers, Anticonvulsants			
Brand Name	**Generic Name**	**Class**	**Daily Dosage Range ***
Depakote	divalproex	anticonvulsant	750mg – 3000mg
Eskalith	lithium carbonate	mood stabilizer	600mg – 2400mg
Gabitril	tiagabine	anticonvulsant	32mg – 56mg
Lamictal	lamotrigine	anticonvulsant	100mg – 200mg
Neurontin	gabapentin	anticonvulsant	900mg – 1800mg
Symbyax	olanzapine/fluoxetine	**	6/25mg – 12/50mg
Tegretol	carbamazepine	anticonvulsant	600mg – 1200mg
Topamax	topiramate	anticonvulsant	200mg – 400mg
Trileptal	oxcarbazepine	anticonvulsant	600mg – 1200mg
* Suggested adult dose ** atypical antipsychotic/antidepressant Note: Dosage ranges may vary depending on source, and may vary according to age.			

CHAPTER 12

Antianxiety Medications, Sleep Agents

Patients being treated for anxiety disorders are often prescribed anti- anxiety or anxiolytic medications. These drugs are often employed in combination with psychotherapy, rendering the individual more susceptible to behavior modification interventions. In addition, the antidepressants discussed in Chapter 8—in particular, the selective serotonin re-uptake inhibitors (SSRIs)—are also used in the treatment of some anxiety disorders, either in combination with a specific anxiolytic or alone.

This Chapter will focus on the main classes of anti-anxiety drugs used to treat the most common anxiety disorders described in Chapter 6. Some of these medications are more effective than others for treating particular disorders, and some may need to be used in combination with SSRIs and other medications, especially in cases of Obsessive- Compulsive Disorder (OCD) and Posttraumatic Stress Disorder (PTSD).

THE ANTI-ANXIETY GROUP

Benzodiazepines act throughout the central nervous system and have muscle relaxation, sedative, anxiolytic and anticonvulsant effects. As a class, they enhance the actions of GABA, which blocks the rapid release of stress hormones associated with anxiety and panic, providing a dissociative or numbing effect on anxiety. The issue of what a user wants these drugs to do and for how long is particularly paramount because psychological or physical dependence concerns lurk in the shadows. Benzodiazepines are more similar than they are different. Prescriber decisions about which benzodiazepine to use are typically based on the anxiety disorder being treated, as well as on the onset of action and rate of elimination of the agent. For example, in the treatment of generalized anxiety disorder, longer half-life benzodiazepines, such as Valium (diazepam) and Klonopin (clonazepam), are often the drugs of choice, due to their longer duration of action.

The term "half-life" refers to the amount of time required for a medication to decrease its concentration by 50 percent relative to its peak level. Those with longer half-lives tend to be eliminated more slowly and therefore can build up in the system, whereas shorter half-life medications are more rapidly excreted leading to less system build up.

Nonbenzodiazepines

In 1960 Librium (chlordiazepoxide) was the first benzodiazepine to reach the U.S. market. Three years later it was followed by Valium (diazepam). Today, benzodiazepines like Xanax (alprazolam) and Ativan (lorazepam) are frequently the drugs of choice for the treatment of panic disorders. That's because they work fast enough to manage the acute symptoms of panic—such as racing pulse and shortness of breath—yet long enough to control the residual anxiety symptoms that typically fuel the concern and worry about future attacks. Benzodiazepines are often used in conjunction with SSRI antidepressants in the treatment of panic. Benzodiazepines, when used short term, can be particularly effective in managing adjustment disorders with anxious mood, such as a recent job loss, death of a close friend or family member, or recent divorce. These medications also treat insomnia and have anticonvulsant properties, relax skeletal muscle, treat alcohol withdrawal and sometimes treat the side effects of antipsychotics.

Whether or not benzodiazepines cause cognitive side effects (verbal learning, speed of thinking, etc.) is controversial. A meta-analysis has concluded that these agents do influence cognitive dysfunction during treatment, and that although cognitive function improved upon discontinuation of the benzodiazepine, it did not return to the level of functioning observed in the control groups not taking benzodiazepines.

Half-Lives of Benzodiazepines and Nonbenzodiazepines	
Half-Life	**Drug**
6 hours or less	Lunesta* (eszopiclone), Halcion (triazolam), Sonata* (zaleplon), Ambien* (zolpidem), Ambien CR*(zolpidem CR), Rozerem* (ramelteon) Edular* (zolpidem tartrate)
8 to 16 hours	Ativan (lorazepam), Restoril (temazepam), Xanax (alprazolam)
More than 24 hours	Valium (diazepam), Dalmane (flurazepam), Librium (chlordiazepoxide), Tranxene (clorazepate)
*nonbenzodiazepine	

Benzodiazepine Advantages

- Very safe in overdose
- Generally, onset of action is quick
- Users are quite compliant with taking them

Benzodiazepine Disadvantages

- All of them influence tolerance and dependence
- Sedative effects can be dangerous when combined with other anxiolytics or central nervous system depressants like alcohol
- Can cause impairment similar to intoxication (slurred speech, poor judgment resulting from inhibition)

Rapid Onset Agents

- Valium (diazepam)
- Tranxene (clorazepate)
- Dalmane (flurazepam)

Intermediate Onset Agents

- Librium (chlordiazepoxide)
- Xanax (alprazolam)
- Ativan (lorazepam)
- Halcion (triazolam)

Slow Onset Agents

- Klonopin (clonazepam)

Physical Dependence Onset Parameters

- Valium (diazepam): 15mg daily for 90 days
- Xanax (alprazolam): 1.5mg daily for 45 days
- Ativan (lorazepam): 6mg daily for 60 days

Withdrawal symptoms of benzodiazepines include: marked anxiety; poor concentration; muscle pain; perceptual disturbances ("a body disconnected from mind" type of experience) and seizures.

Dependence is linked to a marked preoccupation with procuring the drug, concomitant craving, compulsive use tendencies and frequent relapse in spite of repeated, often adverse consequences.

Successful tapering of benzodiazepines should be done very slowly. Strategies are discussed in Appendix VI. Those following a slow, steady withdrawal sequence have the best chance of discontinuing these drugs altogether. Each stage in the tapering process is accompanied by its own attendant challenges with users often reporting that they feel worse each time dosing is decreased. Many believe that when the taper is finally complete they will feel just awful and unable to function. Just the opposite happens, virtually everyone feels better upon discontinuation—free from the constraints of turning over control to a drug to manage anxiety that only they themselves could get under control and free from feeling sedated and having cloudy thought processes.

With regard to OCD, benzodiazepines generally do not possess anti-obsessional properties. Instead, the serotonin antidepressants—such as Prozac (fluoxetine), Zoloft (sertraline), Paxil (paroxetine), Anafranil (clomipramine) and Luvox (fluvoxamine)—are preferentially first-line agents in the treatment of OCD. The inhibitory effects of serotonin help reduce primitive urges which are OCD-like. They are effective in about half of all patients, producing a 50 to 60 percent reduction in symptoms.

OCD is typically treated with higher doses of serotonin antidepressants—as much as two to three times higher than those used to treat depression and other anxiety disorders. Response to medication typically occurs slowly over a period of 8 to 12 weeks. Because OCD requires much higher dosing parameters for serotonin antidepressants to be potentially effective—thereby exacerbating the side effects of excitability and sleep disruption—and since these medications are so slow to deliver, it can be argued that the risks of antidepressant use outweigh the benefits.

A recent development in the treatment of OCD has been the FDA's approval of "Deep Brain Stimulation." This is the first instance that this procedure, which involves the surgical implantation of electrodes deep within the brain to trigger electrical activity, has been approved for use in a psychiatric syndrome. The implants had previously been used to treat movement disorders, most notably Parkinson's disease. The technique is reserved for intractable obsessive-compulsive disorder when conventional management has failed to generate measurable results. Regardless of the treatment modalities employed however, complete symptom remission is rarely if ever attainable. OCD is unfortunately a chronic "disorder of repetition" with a waxing and waning long-term symptom course.

As for PTSD, benzodiazepines may be effective in managing some of the associated clinical symptoms, such as panic attacks and hyperarousal. Also, any of the other prominently utilized psychotropic medication classes— antidepressants, anticonvulsants and antipsychotics—can be employed in PTSD treatment. Depression, anxiety, mood swings and transient psychotic symptoms often accompany PTSD, so any of these medication categories can be helpful. The antihypertensive prazosin (Minipress) at 6mg nightly can be very effective for PTSD-related nightmares and insomnia.

SLEEP AGENTS

Primary insomnia is comprised of three components—difficulty getting to sleep, trouble staying asleep and early morning awakenings. A more apt word for insomnia is sleeplessness and people with chronic sleep difficulties may experience all three of these components. When contemplating a sleep aid, users need to know what they want the drug to do and for how long. And it's worth remembering that insomnia is often transient and may improve within a matter of days without any intervention.

The nonbenzodiazepines Ambien (zolpidem), Sonata (zaleplon) and Lunesta (eszopiclone) are the most commonly used drugs in the treatment of primary insomnia. Some studies suggest that these agents are associated with less dependence and less cognitive impairment than the benzodiazepines. Benzodiazepines are thought to degrade sleep quality over time, leading many users to conclude that their insomnia worsens the longer they use them. These nonbenzodiazepines however, have demonstrated less interference with rapid eye movement (REM) sleep as well as Stage III and IV delta sleep, two of the primary components of sleep architecture, in some users. As such, they are preferentially prescribed for insomnia. When taken responsibly, these so-called "Z" drugs are safe and effective within certain parameters. For example, if someone is grieving an uncomfortable loss or traveling through many time zones, it's quite acceptable to take these hypnotics for a few nights at a time. Months or years of use though, may be an exercise in futility as dosage increases are all but inevitable, ushering in the risk of dependence.

Another zolpidem product is Edular (zolpidem tartrate). Edular (zolpidem tartrate) is merely a brand-name clone of the generically available Ambien (zolpidem). Edular (zolpidem tartrate) is an oral disintegrating preparation, which means it doesn't have to be taken with fluids.

INTERMEZZO: THE MICROMANAGEMENT OF INSOMNIA HAS ARRIVED

Reaffirming the notion that there is indeed a pill for every ill, the U.S. Food and Drug Administration has approved yet another zolpidem product—Intermezzo (zolpidem tartrate sublingual)—for use as needed for the management of insomnia associated with middle-of-the-night awakenings and difficulty returning to sleep. This is the first time the FDA has approved a drug specifically for this indication. The agency warns that Intermezzo (zolpidem tartrate sublingual) should be used only when there are at least four hours of bedtime remaining.

The word *intermezzo* is a term from the musical world—particularly opera—and is defined as a "brief interlude." This is actually a clever brand name for the drug as per its usage indication outlined above; but it's also a dicey concept beckoning misuse. Sublingual administration allows for rapid absorption into the blood stream when placed under the tongue. The recommended and maximum doses of Intermezzo (zolpidem tartrate sublingual) are 1.75mg for women and 3.5mg for men. The recommended dose is lower for women because women excrete zolpidem at a slower rate compared to men.

When it comes to sleep difficulties, if there's a way to mismanage a medication, some people will find it. Concerns regarding Intermezzo (zolpidem tartrate sublingual) use are as follows:

- Some users will ignore the indications and use this drug to help them get to sleep. Why not do so? If the drug helps reinitiate sleep after awakening, why wouldn't it help someone get to sleep in the first place? The problem with taking it to get to sleep is that upon awakening in the middle of the night people will repeat the dose.

- Folks who awaken more than once during the night, say every two hours or so, would likely exceed the maximum dosage recommendations above.

- Those who use regular 5mg or 10mg zolpidem at bedtime and also experience middle-of-the-night awakenings could easily become confused with which of these drugs they're taking and when. This could happen because some prescribers will issue prescriptions for both products to the same person.

- The warning regarding use at least four hours before arising as planned will be violated. Optimally, if one is scheduled to rise at 7am, Intermezzo (zolpidem tartrate sublingual) shouldn't be used after 3am. Those who count on a pill to promote or maintain sleep will ignore time frames; it's that simple.

In 2007, a large National Institute of Health sponsored study concluded that sleeping medication will reduce sleep latency (the time it takes to go from full wakefulness to falling asleep) by about 30 minutes, and that total sleep time will be increased by only 11 minutes. And numerous studies indicate that cognitive behavioral therapy is just as effective as medication and has a more lasting overall benefit.

The side effects of the nonbenzodiazepines are similar to those of the previously discussed benzodiazepines. But Ambien (zolpidem) has been linked to reports of sleepwalking, sleep-eating and sleep-driving behaviors in some users. Ambien (zolpidem) may interfere in some way with the sleep-wake cycle, in that after taking the drug, some users engage in these physical behaviors with no recollection of having done so. The FDA has issued warnings regarding the possibility of this effect in susceptible individuals.

Rozerem (ramelteon) is a non-controlled substance, unlike the benzodiazepines and nonbenzodiazepines. As such, the drug is not linked to abuse or dependence. Rozerem (ramelteon) is "melatonin-like" in that it targets two specific melatonin receptor sites in the brain, thus its sleep-promoting properties. Melatonin's claim is that its influence on the sleep-wake cycle lets our bodies know when it is time to fall asleep and awaken. It is synthesized and released during darkness and natural levels are present in the blood prior to bedtime. Reported common side effects of Rozerem (ramelteon) are drowsiness, fatigue and dizziness.

The newest player in the non-benzodiazepine space is **Belsomra** (suvorexant). It is actually a new chemical formulation in that it does not exert its hypnotic effects by working at GABA, histamine or melatonin receptors. Instead, Belsomra (suvorexant) does its work at orexin receptors. So what is orexin? Orexin is a hormone that regulates the sleep-wake cycle by promoting awareness and wakefulness through stimulation of brain regions involved in arousal and attention. Orexin bonds to nerve receptors in the brain, emitting signals that keep us awake and alert. Belsomra (suvorexant) is an orexin antagonist and therefore blocks the signaling of orexin, preventing it from acting as it usually does, and thus promoting sleep.

In studies comparing Belsomra (suvorexant) users to those taking placebo, those taking Belsomra (suvorexant) got to sleep quicker and spent less time awake throughout the night. Belsomra (suvorexant) is available in 5, 10, 15 and 20mg tablets and is a schedule IV controlled substance—same category as Ambien (zolpidem).

In the aftermath of last year's FDA warnings about "morning after" impairment which resulted in lower dosing recommendations for the so-called "Z" (zolpidem) sleep agents, the FDA requested next-day driving tests to determine a safe dosing range for Belsomra (suvorexant). These tests showed that those taking the 20mg dose were impaired in the morning. For this reason, the recommended dose is 10mg at bedtime, yet the labeling does allow for titration up to 20mg nightly. The most common side effects are sleepiness of course, headache, unusual dreams and dry mouth.

Other than a unique and novel mechanism of action, there's no other particular reason to consider Belsomra (suvorexant) a superior standout. It will serve its purpose as a sleep agent just fine but don't expect it to outshine its "Z" competitors. Users should be clearly informed about the risks of next day driving and warned not to arbitrarily decide to take higher than recommended doses without consulting the prescriber. As of this writing, pricing has not been clearly established, but it's a safe bet to conclude it will be rather expensive.

Another non-benzodiazepine, Buspar (buspirone), is most often used for the treatment of GAD (generalized anxiety disorder). Advantages of Buspar (buspirone) over the benzodiazepines include little if any sedation, no development of tolerance or dependence, and no potentiation effect if used with alcohol. Disadvantages include a slow onset of action and a lack of efficacy, particularly in prior benzodiazepine users. The drug ostensibly exerts its effect on the serotonin system. This is a likely explanation for how slow Buspar (buspirone) can be to take effect. Side effects are typically minimal and include dizziness, headache, nausea, nervousness and agitation.

Antihistamines

This drug class is used primarily to counteract the effects of histamine, a body chemical involved in allergic reactions. But they also can reduce anxiety through their sedative effects and are sometimes used to treat insomnia. If you have ever taken a Benadryl (diphenhydramine), you may know what I mean. Although not FDA- approved for insomnia, antihistamines can help the user get to sleep but not help with early morning awakenings or staying asleep. Antihistamine use may produce a hangover effect or residual grogginess.

Vistaril (hydroxyzine pamoate) and Atarax (hydroxyzine hydrochloride) are two prescription antihistamines that are used to treat insomnia and symptoms of anxiety, nervous tension and allergies. Antihistamines are not associated with a risk of dependency. They typically work within 20–30 minutes and are effective for 4 to 6 hours. Although not habit- forming, tolerance can develop to their sedative and anxiolytic effects requiring dosage increases. Possible side effects include nausea, fatigue, sedation and dizziness.

Beta Blockers

Have you been tapped to offer a toast at the rehearsal dinner of your best friend's wedding? Are you anxious about sitting for that upcoming licensure exam that you've put off for far too long? Do you find yourself dripping with sweat or shaking like a leaf at the mere thought of delivering a presentation to your company's favored client? If so, you're not alone for sure. Performing under pressure where there is something to lose plagues all of us to some extent. If or when you find yourself in such a situation, beta-blocker medications can potentially make quite a bit of difference for the better.

By blocking beta receptors in the heart, blood pressure, heart rate and cardiac output are all decreased. This has led to clinical uses in the treatment of hypertension, angina, and cardiac arrhythmias. Outside of physical medicine though, beta blockers are used in the treatment of anxiety-prone situations with symptoms such as palpitations, sweating and tremor.

Commonly prescribed beta blockers are Inderal (propranolol), Tenormin (atenolol) and Toprol (metoprolol). When taken one to two hours prior to a stressful event, side effects are negligible—possibly a bit of tiredness and a slowed heart rate—which of course is a goal in alleviating peripheral anxiety symptoms. Beta blockers are contraindicated though in those with asthma, emphysema and other respiratory disorders.

Use of Inderal in performance anxiety is customarily in a dosage range of 10–60mg—again to be taken one to two hours prior to the perceived stressful circumstance. These drugs have long benefited performers in many genres appear calm and collected when the "red light" goes on.

Catapres (clonidine)

Also an effective antihypertensive agent, the usefulness of Catapres (clonidine) in the treatment of anxiety is related to its effectiveness in easing some of the peripheral symptoms associated with opiate and alcohol withdrawal, such as tremulousness, profuse sweating, motor restlessness, anxiety and agitation. It can also ease insomnia, due to its sedative effects.

Treating Anxiety with Antipsychotics and Anticonvulsants

The new kids on the block for anxiety management are the second-generation antipsychotics and the anticonvulsants. Use of these agents for anxiety symptoms has been trending for some time now, so let's take a closer look.

As for the atypical antipsychotics, Seroquel XR (quetiapine extended-release) 50 or 150mg per day is getting the most attention. Seroquel XR's (quetiapine extended-release) efficacy is most likely related to its strong antihistamine properties. Although the studies on this drug were industry-funded, the numbers were impressive when compared to placebo as well as to the SSRIs Lexapro (escitalopram) and Paxil (paroxetine). But despite these positive findings, Seroquel XR (quetiapine extended release) has not yet garnered FDA approval for generalized anxiety disorder primarily due to safety factors. This drug requires closer monitoring because of metabolic side effects such as elevated blood sugar, cholesterol and lipid levels.

As for other atypical antipsychotics, Risperdal (risperidone) was no more effective than placebo, and Zyprexa (olanzapine) use as an anxiolytic was plagued by weight gain issues. Other atypical antipsychotics don't even land an honorable mention.

As for the anticonvulsants, they exert their therapeutic action by curtailing excessive neuron activation so their use in anxiety treatment seems logical. That said, only one agent out of a dozen or so shows any benefit for anxiety in randomized trials—and that would be Lyrica (pregabalin) which at doses of 300–600mg per day, can reduce GAD symptoms. Lyrica (pregabalin) also holds its own when compared to the benzodiazepines Ativan (lorazepam) and Xanax (alprazolam) as well as the SNRI antidepressant Effexor (venlafaxine). Despite its apparent effectiveness, Lyrica (pregabalin) is linked to an elevated, dose- dependent risk of sleepiness, dizziness and weight gain. Thus, it continues to be rejected by the FDA for the treatment of generalized anxiety disorder.

When it comes to managing anxiety pharmacologically, the more things change the more they seem to stay the same, because the atypical antipsychotics and the anticonvulsants face more headwinds from a safety perspective. Though effective, Seroquel XR (quetiapine extended- release) and Lyrica (pregabalin) tote along baggage which the benzodiazepines and serotonin antidepressants don't. This baggage weighs down the user of these drugs such that the FDA is erring on the side of caution—particularly for long-term devotees to these drugs.

Side Effects of Anti-anxiety Agents	
Antianxiety Agent	**Side Effects**
Benzodiazepines Examples: Valium (diazepam), Librium (chlordiazepoxide), Xanax (alprazolam), Ativan (lorazepam), Klonopin (clonazepam)	Drowsiness, possible confusion, dizziness, imbalance, potential for physical and psychological dependence. If taken with alcohol, extreme drowsiness and even respiratory depression can occur. Signs of possible overdose include slurred speech and memory problems.
Nonbenzodiazepines Examples: Ambien (zolpidem), Sonata (zaleplon), Lunesta (eszopiclone)	Drowsiness, dizziness, fatigue, sleepwalking, possible interference with REM sleep and sleep/wake cycling. Potential for dependence, withdrawal and tolerance.
Rozerem (ramelteon)	Drowsiness, dizziness, nausea, fatigue, headache, and insomnia. No risk of dependence.
BuSpar (buspirone)	Headache, nausea, dizziness and possible adverse effects on patients with liver or kidney disease. No risk of dependence. No potentiation with alcohol.
Antihistamines Examples: Benadryl (diphenhydramine), Vistaril (hydroxyzine pamoate), Atarax (hydroxyzine hydrochloride)	Drowsiness, fatigue, dry mouth, twitching, tremors.
Beta blockers Examples: Inderal (propranolol), Tenormin (atenolol)	Depression, fatigue, drowsiness, dizziness, lightheadedness, bradycardia (slow heart rate), hypotension (lowered blood pressure). Contraindicated in cases of asthma and emphysema.
Alpha-2 agonist Example: Catapres (clonidine)	Dizziness, drowsiness, postural hypotension (drop in blood pressure when rising quickly from a sitting or lying position), bradycardia (slow heart rate), dry mouth.

CASE STUDY: PANIC DISORDER—"ELEVATOR TO THE 52ND FLOOR"

Philip is a 33-year-old attorney who recently became a full partner in his small law firm. He is married and is the father of two children, ages 3 and 5. He self-referred to you, a Licensed Clinical Social Worker, on the recommendation of a friend you treated two years ago. When you ask Philip why he has decided to see you, he states that two days ago, he and three of his fellow attorneys left their office for a routine business lunch. Upon returning, they boarded the elevator to their office on the 52nd floor. Philip says the elevator moved very slowly, eventually coming to a complete stop between the 51st and 52nd floors. Not overly concerned by this, he was able to call the building maintenance department and alert them of their predicament. Although the maintenance department worked diligently to get the elevator moving again, their attempts were in vain. Philip and his colleagues were trapped in the elevator for more than five hours. They were eventually "welded out" through the elevator's top panel and pulled to safety along the cable structure. Philip stated that although the situation was harrowing, at no point did he "fall apart" or fear for his life. However, since that incident, Philip reports that he has been unable to board any elevator. Upon approaching one, he becomes shaky, lightheaded and short of breath, and he starts to tremble. Philip reports no previous personal or family psychiatric history. His colleagues have allowed him to work from home for now, provided that he seeks treatment.

Diagnostic Considerations

While conducting a thorough assessment of Philip's presenting problem, you ask when he had last seen his primary care physician for a routine physical examination. Philip replies that he visited his physician approximately two months prior to the elevator incident, and that he was found to be in good health. He also explains that he has no personal or family history of psychiatric illness or substance abuse. The discussion then turns to his harrowing circumstances with the elevator.

You mention that although via self-report he had not panicked during the incident itself, he has developed anticipatory anxiety and has understandably become phobic about elevator use. You explain that if these symptoms remain unchecked, the anxiety, fear and subsequent avoidance may potentially worsen. You suggest a psychiatric referral. Philip readily consents.

Treatment Course

The consulting psychiatrist decides to start Philip on Xanax (alprazolam) at 0.25 mg three times daily for management of the associated anxiety. After one week, with Philip's consent, Celexa (citalopram) 20 mg daily is added to the treatment regimen. After two weeks on this regimen, Philip reports feeling markedly less anxious so the psychiatrist begins tapering the Xanax (alprazolam) use, while increasing the Celexa (citalopram) dose to 40 mg daily. As this point, Philip consents to do cognitive-behavioral work. This involves systematic desensitization techniques accompanied by measured exposure to help Philip overcome his elevator phobia. After four months of behavioral work, together with the Celexa (citalopram) use, Philip is consistently able to board and ride the building's elevators up to his 52nd floor office without major incident.

CASE STUDY: OCD "I WANT TO STOP ACTING SO WEIRD"

Douglas is a 46-year-old model maker for a high-tech Fortune 500 company. He was referred to you, a Licensed Professional Counselor, by his parish priest, whom Douglas consulted with for help with anxiety and "behavioral repetition." Douglas tells you that over the last six months, he has found it increasingly difficult to "get out of the house." Douglas mentions that although he has always been a "safety freak" of sorts, some of his recent behavior has been extreme. In recent days, for example, he has returned home as many as 15 times after leaving for work. Each time, he checks the locks on all of the doors and windows, makes sure the appliances are unplugged, and ensures that no water is running from any of the faucets. He also mentions a desire for "order" at his office workspace and says that when a fellow worker stops by and touches or moves something on his desk, Douglas feels annoyed.

In obvious distress, Douglas shares that he feels shame, guilt and increasing self-doubt about all of this. He wants to stop acting "so weird." He also reveals that just last week, his wife asked Douglas for a divorce, saying she could no longer tolerate his "very strange tendencies." Douglas also fears that he is about to be fired from his job. Douglas further reports that his father, a pharmacist, essentially had to retire "in shame" from his work in a retail pharmacy several years ago. The father would repeatedly check the contents of prescription bottles and labels to such an extent that customers complained vehemently about having to wait too long.

Diagnostic Considerations

Having completed your initial assessment, you decide to commend Douglas for having the courage to address these concerns. You inquire about his understanding of OCD and its associated symptoms. He states that he knows little about it, outside of a recent discussion he had listened to on a daytime TV talk show. For explanatory purposes, and to put Douglas at ease, you mention that the disorder has received increasingly more attention over the last few years, that it is considered genetic, and that it is best treated through a combination of medication and behavioral therapies. Douglas consents to begin seeing a psychiatrist colleague of yours who specializes in OCD and has conducted numerous medication clinical trials regarding its management.

Treatment Course

Douglas is started on Paxil (paroxetine) 20 mg daily for one week. In the second week of treatment, the dose is increased to 40 mg daily, and by week three, to 60 mg per day. Throughout the dosage increases, Douglas complains of troubling side effects, including dry mouth, sweating, constipation, and an increasing lack of motivation that he finds particularly troubling. The psychiatrist explains to Douglas that these side effects are consistent with dosage increases, and he recommends ways to best manage them.

Douglas begins to show some initial symptom improvement after six weeks of Paxil (paroxetine) use. But after taking Paxil (paroxetine) at 60 mg per day for three months, Douglas's symptom improvement has essentially plateaued. The atypical antipsychotic Risperdal (risperidone), at a dose of 4 mg per day, is added to the Paxil, and Douglas is instructed to remain on this regimen for another nine months.

From the outset of treatment, you employed a series of "in-vivo response and prevention" cognitive-behavioral techniques to augment medication management. Douglas's symptoms waxed and waned over one year of treatment. Before he leaves treatment, you explain to him that OCD is a chronic disorder for which there is no "cure." Therefore, symptoms tend not to completely remit, but only gradually improve.

Dosage Range Chart—Anti-Anxiety Medications, Sleep Agents			
Brand Name	**Generic Name**	**Class**	**Daily Dosage Range***
Ambien	zolpidem	nonbenzodiazepine	5mg – 10mg
Ativan	lorazepam	benzodiazepine	2mg – 6mg
Belsomra	suvorexant	orexin antagonist	10mg – 20mg
BuSpar	buspirone	nonbenzodiazepine	15mg – 60mg
Dalmane	glurazepam	benzodiazepine	15mg – 60mg
Edular	zolpidem tartrate	nonbenzodiazepine	5mg – 10mg
Halcion	triazolam	benzodiazepine	0.125mg – 0.5mg
Intermezzo	zolpidem sublingual	nonbenzodiazepine	1.75mg – 3.5mg
Klonopin	clonazepam	benzodiazepine	0.5mg – 4mg
Librium	chlordiazepoxide	benzodiazepine	15mg – 100mg
Lunesta	eszopiclone	nonbenzodiazepine	1mg – 3mg
ProSom	estazolam	benzodiazepine	1mg – 2mg
Rozerem	ramelteon	melatonin type	8mg
Sonata	zaleplon	nonbenzodiazepine	5mg – 10mg
Tranxene	clorazepate	benzodiazepine	7.5mg – 60mg
Valium	diazepam	benzodiazepine	5mg – 40mg
Xanax	alprazolam	benzodiazepine	0.5mg – 4mg

*Suggested adult dose

Note: Dosage ranges may vary depending on source, and may also vary according to age.

CHAPTER 13

Anxiety and Insomnia: Treatment Beyond Medication

The least convincing evidence for psychotropic medication use is in the treatment of the anxiety disorders. Here's why: anxiety is as much a cognitive issue as it is an emotional one. Most of us experience anxiety intermittently. It rises to disorder proportions when there is constancy to it, when chronic, anxiety is invariably linked to faulty, irrational or illogical belief systems which require reframing and restructuring to make relief attainable.

The prominent anxiety disorders are Panic Disorder, Generalized Anxiety Disorder, Obsessive Compulsive Disorder and Posttraumatic Stress. Here's a look at each along with a discussion of Insomnia, and what interventions they respond to most favorably sans medication.

Panic Disorder

Panic attacks are sudden, intense, physical and emotional spikes of adrenalin that typically last 10 minutes or so. They rise to disorder proportions when someone hands over control to the panic by worrying excessively about future attacks and avoiding situations that may ignite them.

When treating someone with a history of panic, never initiate treatment from the perspective of their not panicking again. Such an approach is tantamount to telling a kid not to touch anything in Toys "R" Us. Expect that it will happen again and have the client plan accordingly. Explain that they're seeking success, not perfection, and that a step backward serves as a learning experience enabling them to move two or even three steps forward. Remind them that although the physical symptoms of panic are uncomfortable and embarrassing at times, they've survived each and every panic attack they have had, and if they hadn't, well, there wouldn't be a conversation.

Such an approach is the first step toward desensitizing every aspect of the panic situation that could trigger an attack. When suggesting that it's okay to panic, it lowers the stakes, taking the wind out of the sails of panic thus reducing the pressure that clients often place on themselves to keep it from happening again. It's a win-win—if it happens again, it's no big deal, if it doesn't, issue solved.

Another important element of treatment is to reassure the client that they will never likely be able to anticipate every possible trigger of panic. Thus have them prepare to panic and plan how to cope with it. Preparation involves several straightforward steps:

1. **Breathe, breathe, breathe.** It matters not the breathing exercise one utilizes as long as it's done correctly and consistently throughout the day to diminish the adrenalin rush response.

2. **Desensitize.** Let's take the example of someone who is prone to panic when driving on a busy interstate highway: The first step would be to take the next readily available exit and find a safe place to stop the vehicle. The second step would be to place the car in park. The third step would be initiating breathing exercises, popping in a relaxation CD, praying or meditating and imagining a scenario where one is driving along comfortably in control.

3. **Write down the exact steps enumerated in #2 to be taken if or when panic occurs.**

4. **Store it someplace where it's readily available.** Cellphones are great for this as practically everyone has one, particularly when taking to the road.

5. **Do a dress rehearsal via a trial run before resuming normal activity.** The plan here would be to access one short stretch of interstate at off-peak times when it would be easy to get off and get home.

6. **Then take it live under customary circumstances with the understanding that if panic occurs, *a plan is in place, and that plan can be easily and quickly accessed.***

7. **Evaluate.** Commend oneself for having the courage to tackle this; do some self-praise for getting through the situation without panic; decide on what needs changing if results were unfavorable.

8. **Exult.** Irrespective of the outcome, chalk it up as yet another survival.

GENERALIZED ANXIETY DISORDER

Best described as low-level anxiety without panic, GAD is often accompanied by somatic complaints—most often the culprits reported are stomach aches and headaches. GAD is defined by chronic worry in spite of no objective stressors. Faulty beliefs predicated on the "control value" associated with worry keep affected people stuck in a perpetual cycle of rumination.

Cognitive-behavioral reframing work of some type—via any of the widely accepted contemporary models (traditional cognitive-behavioral; dialectical- behavioral; motivational interviewing; mindfulness)—is essential to deescalate the intensity and frequency of worry. Here are four action steps which have stellar track records for addressing and reeling in unbridled worry:

1. **Sort out what is a real problem in the present, what can and cannot be controlled and what's actually doable.** It's interesting that anxious people are often very competent at handling REAL, identifiable problems. This is because an unmistakable problem points us toward a solution path that leaves little if any doubt as to the steps needed to solve it. Here's an example: A client of mine that I am treating for anxiety reported to me that he had all four of his automobile tires stolen. When I inquired as to how this affected him, he stated that after absorbing the initial shock and realizing that he most assuredly wouldn't be recovering the stolen tires, he quickly sprang into action by calling the police, contacting his insurance company, scheduling an appointment with the company's adjuster and purchasing another set of tires. In this example, the man clearly identified what he could control and what he couldn't and acted accordingly. Why? <u>Because a clear plan of action calms the anxious mind, removing any ambiguity as to what needs to be done in the present moment.</u>

2. **Distinguish what is a problem from what might be a problem.** If a person working in a stable job where there have been no layoffs in many years finds himself asking "what if I lose my job," it should be recognized that given the company's history, this is no more than an anxious thought because there is no specific problem to be solved. On the other hand, if this same person has become aware that his company will lay off 30 percent of its workforce within 3 months, then an actual, possible problem exists, and this can be addressed with a plan.

3. **Commit to resolving the worry through planning.** Let's say someone is concerned about a breakdown on the road during a long automobile

trip. In such an instance, it's important to plan for the "what if" and the "what." The "what if" might include recording the phone number of the state police in one's phone, making sure that an AAA membership is current and checking the spare tire before embarking. The "what" (when it happens), would mean actually calling the police or AAA.

4. **Develop a thought-stopping technique and get the body moving.** For someone wishing to push away from worrisome thoughts, instructing themselves to say STOP immediately is a must. This should then be followed up with listening to a meditation CD, an audiobook, singing out loud or conjuring up a healthy, pleasant or even breathtaking image that one has had or would like to experience. But this is not enough. To accelerate the thought-changing process, moving the body is essential. When thought change and physical action are working in unison, it's much harder for the worrier to keep replacing one anxious thought with another and another. Practically any activity can work. If at home, examples are cleaning the house, doing a load of laundry, taking a walk outside or tending to a pet. At work, walking around the desk or up and down a couple of flights of stairs while thinking about the work task at hand can be most helpful.

Biological constructs as well as life experiences shape anxiety—even when there is no objective evidence that something is clearly wrong or is a problem. In this vein, a threatening situation and its accompanying thoughts are always lurking around in search of a subject. The good news is that this is not only manageable, but in many cases solvable. And just maybe one of the best strategies of all is to take a lighthearted approach to anxiety and laugh at it when in its grip.

OBSESSIVE-COMPULSIVE DISORDER

An apt description of OCD is that it manifests as a cycle of excessive carefulness. OCD-affected people can be very exacting, meticulous and fastidious— invoking anger and frustration from those living and working within their daily sphere. Symptoms often emerge during childhood or early adolescence and unfortunately remain stable if left untreated.

As an avid blogger and publisher of a monthly newsletter, I get questions – many, many questions. Here's one regarding OCD:

"I am adamant about toilet tissue being placed on the roller so that the tissue dispenses from the top of the roll, not the bottom. When other family place it on

the roller in reverse, I become irritated and immediately change it back." "Does this mean I have OCD?"

My answer: "No, unless you're guarding the roller all day as if you were a sentinel keeping watch."

We all have preferences which can manifest as eccentricities, oddities or habits. The key is to what extent does our way of doing things affect our personal, social or occupational functioning. OCD is a baffling son-of-a-gun of a disorder. In the literature, it has been referred to as "the full-time companion." The phrase I've coined for it is "a disorder of excessive carefulness accompanied by an exaggeration of possible danger."

The hallmark presentation is thought and behavior-driven. Initial inquiries for treatment, in my experience, come most often from spouses and other family.

So, what's the basis for these seemingly odd thought and behavior occurrences? The most salient, plausible explanation I can offer goes like this: When we humans recognize danger, there is a trigger switch embedded in the basal ganglia which flips into the "on" position. Then, as we begin the process of resolving this danger, the switch transitions to "dimmer" mode and then to the "off" position—with successful resolution. For example, let's say you are preparing breakfast and after having done so, you forget to turn off the stove. You may recognize this by the sizzling that continues in the cooking pan, the heat coming from the cooktop, or you may see the flame itself. So, you switch the stove control knob to the off position, check it once or twice, and proceed with your day. Your trigger switch came on, then dimmed, and moved to off as you snuffed out the potential danger.

The OCD sufferer's switch unfortunately doesn't cycle, remaining perpetually in the "on" mode. Thus, their instincts are out of control and they cannot reel in primitive urges and behaviors. As such, OCD may begin as a result of a precipitating event—but not always.

Getting better is best approached by addressing what doesn't work—and that would be a "logical" approach. Yet logic is precisely what loved ones tend to employ in an attempt to help. A statement like "the car door is locked, you've checked it several times" results in abject failure. OCD affected people know the door is locked, but that doesn't ameliorate the safety threat. Treatment professionals understand that the threat remains alive in spite of the constant checks and that the repetitiveness of the checking rituals becomes increasingly unnerving. So they work backwards by addressing the ritualistic behaviors first, understanding that as response prevention increases, the intensity of the obsessions will diminish. This strategy is referred to as ERP—exposure and response prevention. Let's take the example of someone with "germophobia." Treatment may resemble something like this: clean the bathtub with gloves at first, gradually reducing the incidence of hand washing after cleaning; then progressively work toward cleaning without gloves and without excessive hand washing. The goal is to get the individual to obsess less about becoming contaminated.

I also employ the strategy outlined in the previous section, but with a twist. I'll have the affected individual write himself "fan mail" in advance of treatment—which outlines the changes he has announced he wants to make. I've found this to be an effective way for him to push himself to take the steps that actually generate the actions necessary for goal attainment. And where applicable, I'll have him take photos of the situation that is generating so much concern. For the checker who fears that the stove is still on in spite of objective evidence to the contrary, I'll have him snap a close-up image of the knobs in the "off" position. I'll have him print the photo and attach his fan mail as a caption—"my stove is off and I can see that is; I choose to believe what I see, and I enjoy feeling relieved." Then I will have him post the photo and look at it several times a day. This type of intervention can also be generalized to excessive hand washing, a need for symmetry or order and hoarding manifestations of OCD.

OCD is not only baffling, it's mysterious also. Those with the disorder tend to pick their poison. Rarely do I encounter a chronic checker who is also a chronic hand washer, thus blurring the lines regarding the recognition of danger. Safety concerns don't necessarily correlate with contamination concerns.

Success with OCD is best defined by the extent of symptom reduction. Complete eradication of symptoms is unattainable and therefore an irrational and illogical goal. With ongoing improvement, people with OCD often develop considerable insight into the disorder. They gradually come to understand that these symptoms are a part of them and help define their uniqueness. With this in mind, they then give themselves permission to have the symptoms and adapt to them. OCD also seems to improve with age thereby providing long-term hope for those affected by this often humiliating syndrome.

POSTTRAUMATIC STRESS DISORDER

Engaging the PTSD-affected individual in behavioral therapies is paramount. Symptom improvement is contingent upon two factors: (1) making the fight-or-flight response come to an end; and (2) helping the identified individual to better utilize their imagination to create new, healthier realities. The eventual goal is to move the individual to the present as opposed to continuing to view life through the lens of the trauma. Here are a couple of strategies to consider:

- **Cognitive-behavioral and Exposure Therapy.** Cognitive-behavioral therapies that employ Dialectical behavioral and Mindfulness techniques help alter behavior through dialogue that assists the patient in recognizing the maladaptive connections between their thoughts and emotions. Exposure therapy involves confronting patients over and over with what is haunting them, gradually introducing desensitization.

- **Eye Movement Desensitization and Reprocessing (EMDR).** An example of an often employed EMDR technique has a clinician wiggling fingers back and forth across a patient's field of vision with the patient tracking the fingers while holding the traumatic memories in mind. Proponents claim that the technique enables patients to process their traumas such that they fade into memories and stop affecting the present.

Any therapy that helps patients better tolerate their bodily sensations and aids them in becoming more adept at processing the trauma themselves can be helpful. Yoga can be especially effective at doing this as is also the case with tapping techniques. With the tapping technique, under a therapist's direction, a patient taps various acupressure points with his or her own fingertips. If done correctly, it can calm the sympathetic nervous system and prevent the patient from being thrown into fight-or-flight mode.

INSOMNIA

Infants can sleep anywhere. As a frequent flyer, I notice this often. In spite of the hustle and bustle of getting the passengers onboard and the roar of jet engines upon takeoff, little ones find dreamland, often safely tucked away in the arms of a loved one. Sleep though is not a birthright and this can become painfully obvious as we age.

The first step to attaining reasonably sound, restful sleep is to do an assessment of one's life circumstances. Think possible physical causes first. What about breathing difficulty or sleep apnea? Is pain an issue? How about restless legs? Significant advances in pharmacotherapy render all of these conditions readily treatable, so physician consultation is the next right step. Then, what about certain medications that may be promoting wakefulness?

Caffeine is a drug, and nasal decongestants for sinus or allergy conditions often contain ingredients which will slow sleep onset. How about alcohol use prior to bedtime? Alcohol adversely affects Delta or deep sleep. Next, consider what's going on between the ears. What's on your mind when your head hits the pillow at night? Is it the same issue or a number of different concerns? What is short-circuiting the resolution of these issues? Bedtime is not conducive to worrying about wayward children or cracking the code to a better relationship with an obtuse boss. Time should be set aside during the day to address these and other troublesome issues when more alert.

Then there's the prickly issue of sleep sabotage. Here's a short list for delaying an appointment with the sandman:

1. **Anything with an "I:" I-phones, I-pads, I-pods, I-tunes.**
2. **A light-filled sleeping space.**
3. **Room temperature.**
4. **A heavy meal.**
5. **Alcohol, caffeine, decongestants.**
6. **Stimulating movies (Halloween, Nightmare on Elm Street and The Exorcist are way up there).**

Sleep induction, on the other hand is conducive to the following:

1. **If it has an On/Off switch, choose "Off" at least 30 minutes before bedtime.** This means rounding up the usual suspects—the TV, the "I" culprits listed above and any other device that falls in the technology category. It's impossible to wind down with these devices, talking, singing, humming, beeping or ringing.
2. **Set the sleeping room temperature at a level comfortable for you, ideally somewhere between shivering and sweating.** This means negotiating with a spouse or partner to find a set point somewhere between a meat locker and a sauna. Lots of wiggle room here.
3. **Pray, meditate or read something soothing (a gentle romance novel) or boring (the U.S. Tax Code).** Repetitive prayer is a great sleep inducer; meditation CDs or exercises relax the mind; reading something that is non-stimulating tires us cognitively.
4. **Take all medication one hour before bedtime.** The last thing you need after getting to sleep is a bathroom interruption. As we age, not

only does the Sandman greet us with more folded arms, it's also more challenging to retain fluids we've consumed around bedtime without often frequent trips to the water closet. Restricting fluids after eating dinner is a good idea for most of us; this is not the time to hydrate—thus the one-hour rule for medication consumption.

5. **Tire the mind and the body.** Tiring the mind is generally the easier of the two. Getting through the workday means focusing, studying or concentrating on the task at hand. This helps us get to sleep. Tiring the body means moving the body, helping us stay asleep. Tiring the body requires a different type of exercise—something the body doesn't adapt to naturally—engendering resistance to physical workouts. <u>Nevertheless, this is the ONLY way to effectively help us stay asleep.</u> Brisk walking and yoga are two excellent choices.

6. *If you do nothing else,* **get the sleeping room as dark as possible.** This helps stimulate the secretion of melatonin, a naturally occurring sleep hormone.

While we sleep, the brain transforms our day's experiences into memories and learning and releases hormones that fuel growth, build muscle mass and repair tissue. Sleep also releases hormones that fight infections and influence diet and weight.

Science has yet to uncover why we need sleep, so it's best to just accept that we do and to get plenty of it.

SPECIFIC POPULATIONS, ADHD, HERBALS & SUPPLEMENTS, SOLVING MEDICATION CHALLENGES

CHAPTER 14

Specific Population Groups

Pregnancy

Physicians have been understandably reluctant to prescribe psychotropic medications to women who are either pregnant or contemplating pregnancy. For one, there is the paucity of reliable data associated with their use. For another, there are unknown risks to the fetus. Also, few women would intentionally place their unborn child at possible risk by using psychiatric medications while pregnant.

However, nearly half of all pregnancies are unplanned, and significant numbers of women of childbearing age are taking medications for anxiety, depression, schizophrenia, bipolar disorder and other psychiatric conditions. This means that a considerable number of women are becoming pregnant at the same time they are being treated for a mental illness. This population must be informed, to the degree possible, of the risks of taking these drugs during pregnancy and nursing.

Despite the lack of extensive data, evidence-based information from epidemiologic studies indicates that most psychotropic drugs are relatively safe during pregnancy. But as it will be explained below, no psychotropic is without at least some risk, with some considered downright unsafe and off limits. Also, there is another issue to consider: Failing to treat pregnant women with a psychiatric diagnosis may be far riskier than the possible drawbacks and complications to the woman or child if psychotropic medications were employed during pregnancy. For example, stopping medications for a woman with a serious illness, such as schizophrenia or bipolar disorder, could trigger a relapse that might endanger both the woman and her baby (poor self care, inadequate nutrition, poor prenatal and antenatal care). Still, it's understandable for expectant mothers and physicians alike to be apprehensive about the use of psychiatric medications during pregnancy. The most important indicator of a healthy baby is a healthy mother.

Safety issues for both mother and child are of paramount importance, so important risk factors linked to drug use during pregnancy should be addressed. A major risk is teratogenesis, or birth defects involving the malformation of the fetus or fetal organs. Teratogenesis is often a result of neural tube defects, where the brain and spinal cord fail to fuse together properly. Spina bifida, or "cleft spine," is a common example. Two other teratogenic manifestations are facial deformity and cleft palate. Drugs that produce these malformations are known as teratogens.

Then there is behavioral teratogenesis—defined as the long-term effects on the child resulting from drug exposure *in utero*. These effects can manifest as learning difficulties and developmental delays. Also, more information has surfaced on the subject of poor neonatal adaptation, defined as residual effects on the newborn that can include such symptoms as hypothermia (low body temperature), difficulties with eating and sleeping, tachycardia (rapid heartbeat) and irritability.

With some exceptions, psychiatric medications generally fall into FDA category C—meaning potential fetal risk cannot be ruled out. All psychiatric medications cross the placental barrier and all are secreted in breast milk.

Antidepressants

Depression is a common phenomenon during pregnancy with between 10–15 percent of pregnant women meeting criteria for major depression and up to 70 percent reporting some symptoms throughout the pregnancy term. Postpartum depression is the most prevalent complicating event, occurring in about 15 percent of women, on average.

Untreated or unrecognized depression is significantly associated with poor pregnancy outcomes. Premature birth rates are higher and the risks of low birth weight infants, as well as postnatal complications, are increased. Also depression that goes unmanaged is linked to an increased tendency to self-medicate with tobacco and drugs with abuse potential, including alcohol.

Psychotherapy is the best initial step for addressing mild or moderate depression during pregnancy. And women reluctant to consent to antidepressants are prime candidates for any of the commonly employed psychosocial therapies utilized today.

When it comes to antidepressant or other psychotropic medication use during pregnancy, the best approach is to begin with conducting a thorough history. The key issue is determining the acuity of the pregnant woman's risk for the occurrence of depressive episodes during childbearing. Fetal exposure to psychotropics and the possibility of depression relapse are vital considerations.

If the risk of relapse is high, warranting the use of medication, discussing pros and cons with the pregnant woman is imperative. The goal of medication management is to establish and maintain a euthymic state throughout the duration of the pregnancy—utilizing the lowest possible effective medication dosing strategies.

Determining risk beckons that certain questions be asked. Some of these include: How serious were previous depressive events? Did treatment, if any, include antidepressants or other psychiatric medications? Was there evidence of postpartum depression, and if so, what were the ramifications? Is the woman currently using psychotropics and for how long? Do they seem to be working? If the medications were discontinued, what happened? Is suicide possibly an issue?

Lastly, the use of multiple medications during pregnancy is a risky proposition. More medications equal a more complicated and potentially more serious adverse events profile, so optimizing and maximizing the benefits of a single medication is the safest and most reasonable strategy. Pregnancy is not the time for testing the waters of experimentation. The best case scenario is that if a woman needs a psychotropic medication during pregnancy and is taking a drug that seems to be working, she should continue on it, until adverse circumstances signal a reevaluation.

According to recent data, none of the antidepressants that have been studied in pregnancy have been found to increase the baseline rate of 1 percent to 3 percent for major fetal malformations. Some studies, however, report an increased rate of spontaneous abortions. The SSRIs, as well as most of the cyclics are not associated with teratogenesis. Past epidemiologic studies have shown an association between first- trimester antidepressant use and congenital cardiac defects, but a *New England Journal of Medicine* study conducted between the years 2000 and 2007 found that the risk of cardiac defects was no higher for depressed women taking SSRIs or other antidepressants than for those who didn't, when controlling for other risk factors. (Study limitations included prescription records which were unable to determine whether the women studied actually took the medication, and information regarding miscarriages and pregnancy termination, which may be a ramification of fetal cardiac defects). During 2006, reports indicated that as many as 30 percent of children with third trimester exposure to SSRIs showed withdrawal: lack of crying, increased muscle tone, irritability and poor sleep.

The MAOIs, Remeron (mirtazapine), Effexor (venlafaxine) and Wellbutrin (bupropion) have not been studied extensively. Antidepressants are present, to some extent, in breast milk; therefore, nursing is generally contraindicated for women taking these drugs.

Lithium is generally not recommended during pregnancy. Its use has been linked to neonatal effects, including impaired respiration and EKG and heart-rate abnormalities. Exposure in the first trimester is strongly associated with fetal cardiac irregularities. Lithium is also linked to Ebstein's anomaly, a heart defect in which the tricuspid valve malfunctions. Lithium is highly concentrated in breast milk; therefore, nursing is contraindicated for women taking this drug.

Antipsychotics

Of all the antipsychotic medications, Haldol (haloperidol) is the agent that has been most studied. Haldol (haloperidol) is not linked to congenital malformations during the first trimester. Therefore, it remains the preferred antipsychotic for use during pregnancy. The newer, second-generation antipsychotics have not been sufficiently investigated so as to determine their safety during pregnancy. All second-generation antipsychotics carry a risk for metabolic syndrome but are associated with less risk for movement disorders—compared to their first-generation counterparts.

Benzodiazepines

Although there is insufficient evidence to prove that benzodiazepines are teratogens, many believe that the use of this class of drugs should be avoided during the first trimester of pregnancy, due to a risk of orofacial clefts. A significant concern with benzodiazepine use during pregnancy is the emergence of neonatal CNS depression and withdrawal symptoms. Other symptoms of abrupt discontinuation syndrome include sedation, hypotonia (loss of muscle tonicity), apnea, reluctance to suck and cyanosis. Benzodiazepines are secreted in breast milk and can cause sedation and slowed heart rate.

Anticonvulsants

Tegretol (carbamazepine) and Depakote (divalproex sodium) are established human teratogens. They should both be avoided during pregnancy. These drugs are also linked to long-term neurodevelopmental effects in offspring well into adolescence, such as EEG pattern changes, expressive language and developmental delays, and intellectual performance deficits. Information on the newer anticonvulsants that has recently come to light is more promising. Specifically, Lamictal (lamotrigine), Trileptal (oxcarbazepine) and Neurontin (gabapentin), when used during pregnancy, do not increase the risk of major birth malformations.

OLDER ADULTS: AN OVERVIEW

Safe medication use in an aging population requires vigilance. Patients and their caregivers must keep track of the quantity and type of medications, making sure they are taken properly and regularly, and watching for any adverse side effects and interactions. These challenges are related to the very real physiological factors that clinicians face when prescribing and administering medications to older adults.

Dosing concerns arise with the elderly. Body weights change, metabolism slows and stomachs do not absorb substances as well as they once did. Kidneys and livers don't process fluids and toxins as efficiently—there can be as much as a 40 percent reduction in the clearance of certain drugs. In post-menopausal women in particular, fatty tissue increases, which can raise the concentrations of certain drugs. Older people also tend to have proportionally less body water, so blood levels of a water-soluble drug can also be higher than would be expected.

Also, the elderly generally take more medications, and tend to "self-medicate" with over-the-counter drugs and herbal supplements more than younger adults. This increases the possibility of drug interactions.

Some estimates place the incidence of drug interactions at 6 percent in patients taking two medications a day—and as high as 50 percent in those taking five a day.

MENTAL ILLNESS IN OLDER ADULTS

With a rapidly aging population, prescribers and non-prescribers alike will no doubt be seeing more elderly patients as more and more Baby Boomers approach retirement. Currently in the United States, those 65 years of age and older make up 13 percent of the total population, but account for 30 percent of all prescriptions written.

An important starting point is the recognition that most mental health syndromes improve with age. Surveys regarding quality of life issues such as happiness and contentment in older adults consistently yield higher scores when compared to people in their midlife years and young adulthood. The obvious exception here would be the neurocognitive disorders which must be controlled for in any quality studies or surveys.

When psychiatric illness does emerge in late life though, the potential ramifications can be significant. So when an elderly individual begins alluding to appetite or sleep problems or is speaking of feeling depressed, we must pay attention.

A viable indicator for when an older person may benefit from more focused psychiatric attention is their ability to thrive. This includes an assessment of activities of daily living—specifically, are they physically mobile, are they able to keep up with daily chores such as getting to the grocery store, managing their finances and safely able to operate an automobile? And if the person is being treated for certain physical disorders, it's essential that this treatment not be segregated from the psychiatric help, because the two may very well be joined together. For example, an elderly woman who complains of feeling listless and dysphoric may very well be experiencing depression, but that depression may be influenced by her history of congestive heart failure and a recent hip replacement. As such, overall infirmity is an important consideration.

When it comes to mood disorders in the elderly, what's most significant is their capacity to experience pleasure. When this waxes and wanes, instead of describing themselves as depressed, they will allude to an increasing lack of interest in seeing their children or grandchildren or even other longtime companions. This is often fueled by a growing lack of patience with others and can influence an increased tendency to socially isolate.

Medicating psychiatric concerns in older adults should be approached with reasonable caution. The time-honored adage of "start low and go slow" takes on much significance when the various psychotropic medication classes are employed. As a general rule, the starting dose should be at least 50 percent of that typically employed in younger, psychiatrically-disordered individuals. Although an older adult may very well need and benefit from higher dosing, beginning medication treatment in this fashion can give rise to intolerable side effects and may exacerbate drug-drug interactions eventually leading to resistance to future use.

Changes in mental status can be drug-related. Benzodiazepines can cause drowsiness, confusion, prolonged sedation and memory loss. All of the antidepressants routinely prescribed in younger age groups are applicable in the elderly. Cyclic antidepressants like Elavil (amitriptyline) though, can cause confusion, and even delirium, when used in the elderly. For sleep problems, trazodone use at 50mg or less is a safe option because of the general absence of anticholinergic effects such as dry mouth, blurred vision, constipation and memory problems. Benzodiazepines and cyclic antidepressants have historically been linked to falls and various types of fractures.

Antipsychotics are currently the most significantly debated medication class when it comes to use in the elderly. When to use them and in what particular setting has become a hot button issue. Many states vigorously enforce and even prohibit their use in nursing home patients, complicating the conundrum as to how to best pharmacologically manage very agitated older folks residing in these facilities. When utilized, the newer, second-generation agents are preferred.

Watch for signs of noncompliance. It sometimes takes longer to see a therapeutic effect with psychotropic medications used in seniors, placing them at risk for abruptly discontinuing their medications due to slowed response rates. Advancing age is often accompanied by less patience. Older adults should be encouraged to continue to take their medications unless otherwise instructed by their physician or other prescriber. Memory often declines with age, too. Encourage patients to keep an updated list of medications with them at all times and provide a copy to a family member.

Elderly patients may be getting their prescriptions from more than one pharmacy. Encourage them to use only one source for the purchase of all medications—prescription and over-the-counter. Pharmacies now have computer software that can check for potentially problematic drug interactions.

Watch for additional medications prescribed to alleviate the side effects of an already prescribed one. For example, a sleep aid may be prescribed to offset the side effect of insomnia from an antidepressant. This can set up a vicious cycle of polypharmacy, a growing and potentially serious concern in the elderly.

It's worth noting that there is good data supporting the use of cognitive-behavioral therapies in conjunction with medication to relieve psychiatric symptoms in this population group. Seniors are usually cooperative and willing to work with more than one discipline. Getting and keeping them connected with more than one treatment professional is the major obstacle, particularly if they are living alone.

Interventions to promote successful aging include an emphasis on physical activity to maintain strength and endurance and reduce the risk of falls. Nutritional strategies include caloric restriction to promote weight loss and increase mobility or the use of supplements to enhance weight gain in those who have lost interest in eating. Also, reducing social isolation through group activities and embracing a sense of spirituality can help considerably.

CHILDREN AND ADOLESCENTS

Age is not a factor when it comes to psychiatric disorder emergence and the psychiatric clinical communities of the world reliably agree on this.

But with the notable exception of psychostimulant use in ADHD, there remains a paucity of reliable data addressing psychopharmacology in children and adolescents. Here are some of the headwinds treating clinicians face:

1. Many medications are rapidly metabolized by children and have greater renal clearance, generally up to puberty. This gives rise to dosing issues. How much is too much, particularly in young children, to produce toxic effects vs. how much is too little to produce therapeutic effects?

2. The role that neurotransmitter development plays in drug response rates remains very unclear. Do children's neuronal systems manufacture serotonin, norepinephrine, and dopamine at different rates than in adults? Much is unknown here.

3. For mood disorders in particular, there is the nature vs. nurture controversy, raising the question as to what extent depression in children is biological vs. environmental vs. both.

4. Co-occurring disorders in children are the rule rather than the exception. Distilling a veritable hodge-podge of symptoms down to something clear-cut is all but impossible. This hinders and further complicates the development of clear rationale for medication use.

5. Youth are targets for diagnostic fads. ADHD was the first fad diagnosis out of the gate in the '80s and early '90s. Bipolar disorder in youth is the most recent fad and autism is gaining. These fads have fueled a veritable explosion of psychotropic medication use in youth which is FDA unapproved.

6. Warnings such as the increased risk of suicidal tendency in children taking antidepressants steer parents away from getting such prescriptions filled and hamstrings prescribers. Thus children who could be helped by antidepressants will never swallow even the first pill.

7. The overall safety vs. efficacy conundrum issue weighs heavily on prescribing practices and has parents and caretakers wondering whether treatment may prove to be more complicated and even worse than the presenting problem.

8. Children are more sensitive to the side effects of psychotropics due to metabolism issues, lack of body mass and undeveloped adaptability skills.

There are no quick and easy solutions to any of these issues. Youth are naturally vulnerable and need to be protected to the fullest extent from predatory medication administration. As such, any significant, measurable advances in medicating psychiatrically disturbed children should continue to progress rather slowly.

Assessing Children and Adolescents

When evaluating children and adolescents for treatment, consider all of the following as part of the assessment process:

1. Whenever possible, observe the child in multiple milieus. For example, children may behave different in social situations when compared to their actions in school or at home.

2. Obtain input from collateral sources (teacher, coach, child care provider) to help confirm what you observe. Assessing and evaluating children appropriately is a team effort.

3. Conduct extensive interviews with the affected child and at least one parent. Children respond to cues and exercises, which although important, may not be enough to confirm your findings. Responsible parents are your de-facto specialists as they observe, interact and listen to the child every day.

4. Do a thorough review of the child's medical history. Undiagnosed medical disorders may be driving the undesirable behaviors exhibited by some children. In general, think in terms of ruling out medical issues first, but particularly do so when the child's behavior is violating the rights of others or accepted social norms.

5. Obtain a thorough family history of psychiatric disorder. Co-occurring conditions are the rule rather than the exception when assessing children, so genetic predisposition issues can potentially be a major ally for you.

Children and Mood Disorders

Depression

According to the National Mental Health Association, one in three American children—some of pre-school age—suffer from depression. Because children and adolescents tend not to spontaneously report symptoms, we often need to rely on observations from parents or primary caretakers.

Signs and symptoms of pediatric depression include:

- Persistent sadness
- Lack of energy, motivation or enthusiasm
- Changes in sleep or eating patterns (too much or too little)
- Irritability, agitation and unwarranted crying
- Developmental delays in language or walking
- Inappropriate, sad or morbid play that concentrates on harming themselves or others and
- Boredom and school failure

According to the NIMH, approximately one in 20 teens has moderately severe to severe major depression, making major depression one of the most common disorders of adolescence. It occurs in both boys and girls and a substantial number of them have suicidal thoughts.

Medicating Depression in Children and Adolescents

Cyclic antidepressants have been used for years in young people. The FDA has approved their use in children at least 12 years of age. The prototype cyclic antidepressant has been Tofranil (imipramine). It has been prescribed for the treatment of Attention Deficit Hyperactivity Disorder (ADHD), school-phobia, night terrors, sleepwalking disorder and enuresis (bedwetting). However, cyclic antidepressants can be dangerous in overdose and are fraught with potentially serious side effects. Six cases of sudden death due to suspected cardiac arrhythmias have been reported in children using Norpramin (desipramine).

The selective serotonin reuptake inhibitors (SSRIs) are considered first-line agents for the treatment of pediatric depression. Although clinical studies are sparse, they illustrate that SSRIs are better tolerated and more effective than the cyclics.

All antidepressants on the U.S. drug market carry an FDA "black box" warning on the labeling, stating a possible risk of suicide when used by children and adolescents. Clinicians face uncertainty regarding the use of antidepressants, especially in youth under the age of eighteen. There is evidence that suicidal ideation may emerge during the early phases of treatment with antidepressants. There is no evidence though that this increases the risk of completed suicides. (No suicides in 4000+ children in any of these studies).

Bipolar Disorder

The assessment and diagnosis of bipolar disorder in youth remains very controversial. Many diagnoses nowadays are made by primary care physicians with little expertise in psychiatry. Also, because of time constraints that accompany a busy primary care setting, primary care doctors typically spend less time with each child, when compared to the amount of time allocated in a more traditional psychiatric setting. There is also little if any consensus on how to effectively manage symptom severity. These factors, particularly over the last decade, have contributed to a diagnostic rush to judgment, pushing pediatric bipolar disorder to fad status. Many kids getting this diagnosis present primarily with temper tantrums and irritability, with classic bipolarity features being largely ignored. This pushes the boundaries of pediatric bipolar disorder far into unconventional territory.

Enter Disruptive Mood Dysregulation Disorder (DMDD), a new diagnosis included in the DSM-5, which essentially creates a less threatening diagnostic haven for kids misdiagnosed as bipolar. There is no credible research on DMDD. It has not been adequately studied, and it is an untested diagnosis. It runs the risk of serving merely as a diagnostic dumping ground for temperamental, yet essentially normal kids who are going through a developmental stage they will eventually outgrow and should not have been diagnosed with any disorder in the first place.

The truth is that bipolar disorder is quite difficult to diagnose in children. Many of its characteristic symptoms overlap with other disorders, particularly ADHD. Irritability, agitation and non-episodic temper outbursts are symptoms not only of ADHD, but also of oppositional defiant disorder, conduct disorder or other anxiety disorders in children. Adding DMDD to this differential mix means that achieving diagnostic accuracy, or getting closer to it, will be even more confounding.

It's true that difficult to manage children are the source of much consternation to parents, teachers and even other children. Thus eager and overly enthusiastic clinicians often feel pressured to please worried parents by diagnosing and treating a child—even in instances where it is not yet possible to make a diagnosis or pursue a safe and efficacious treatment. In such instances, the misdiagnosed ill is so often accompanied by a pill—the subject of the next section.

Medicating Children and Adolescents with Bipolar Disorder

The most widely used medications within the mood stabilizer category for treating pediatric bipolar disorder are lithium and Depakote (divalproex).

Although numerous studies confirm that these medications are effective, their safety is questionable, due to the potential life-long nature of bipolar disorder. Long-term lithium use has been linked to quite a few side effects, ranging from acne and cloudy thinking to weight gain, tremors, decreased thyroid function and kidney problems. As a result, children taking lithium should have their blood levels monitored several times a year. Similarly, long-term use of Depakote (divalproex) can cause liver problems and toxicity. Depakote's (divalproex) potential health risks prompted the FDA to order a "black box" warning to be placed on the medication for both pancreatitis and liver failure. For this reason, any child or adolescent taking Depakote (divalproex) should have blood work every three to six months.

Second-generation antipsychotics also appear to be effective at managing the severe mood swings associated with bipolar disorder in children and teens. But again, benefit-vs.-risk is a concern. These drugs can induce weight gain, sleepiness, parkinsonian and extrapyramidal symptoms, elevated lipid levels, and an increased risk of developing Type II diabetes.

The safety/effectiveness conundrum associated with mood stabilizers and the newer antipsychotics in the treatment of pediatric bipolar disorder will linger until a new, safer generation of compounds is developed. When it comes to treating children, the balance needs to favor minimizing risks. However, for children with serious and potentially dangerous behavioral problems associated with bipolar disorder, the benefits of medication use typically outweigh these risks.

Anxiety Disorders

According to the National Mental Health Information Center, anxiety disorders are among the most common mental, emotional and behavioral problems occurring during childhood and adolescence. About 13 out of every 100 children and adolescents 9 to 17 years of age experience some kind of anxiety disorder, with girls affected more than boys. If left untreated, these disorders can lead to the inability to finish school, impaired social relations, low self-esteem, and eventually, anxiety disorders in adulthood.

The onset of childhood anxiety usually begins between the ages of 6 and 8. Children at this age typically become less afraid of the dark and other imaginary dangers, and they become more afraid and anxious about performance in school and interactions with friends. Some studies suggest that anxiety disorders in children are heritable, particularly from parents meeting anxiety disorder criteria themselves. But there is no way to prove whether the disorders are a result of biology, the environment, or both.

Here is a brief description of types of anxiety disorders diagnosable in children and adolescents:

Generalized Anxiety Disorder: This is similar to adult generalized anxiety disorder (GAD). Children and adolescents with this disorder engage in unrealistic and extreme worry about almost everything—their academic performance, athletic capability, even punctuality. Tense, self-conscious and having a strong desire for reassurance, these young people may complain about aches and pains that have no physical cause.

Panic Disorder: In children and young teenagers, panic is rare. Rates do begin to increase in older adolescents, particularly girls. As they can for adults, repeated panic attacks can be a sign of panic disorder. These attacks may be accompanied by symptoms that include a pounding heartbeat, dizziness, nausea, and feelings of imminent harm or death, accompanied by intense fear.

Separation Anxiety Disorder: In DSM-IV-TR, this disorder was classified under the "Disorders Usually First Diagnosed in Infancy, Childhood or Adolescence" section. And while DSM-IV-TR specified onset before the age of 18, DSM-5 specifies <u>no</u> specific age of onset. In order to meet criteria, fear, anxiety or avoidance must be present for at least four weeks in children and adolescents. In DSM-5, Separation Anxiety Disorder is no longer thought of as a syndrome rooted exclusively in childhood.

Other Disorders Separately Classified in Children and Adolescents

Obsessive-Compulsive Disorder: Like OCD-affected adults, children and adolescents with OCD become trapped in patterns of repetitive thoughts and actions that are difficult to stop. These actions may include repeated hand washing, counting, hair pulling, nail biting, repetitive questioning, arranging and rearranging objects and a strong need to control others and their environment. Children and adolescents often have much higher rates of aggressive obsessions, such as thoughts of harming themselves or others, and sexually acting out. Childhood and adolescent OCD is highly co-morbid with mood, anxiety, tic and disruptive behavior disorders.

The National Institute of Mental Health (NIMH) suggests that nearly 10 percent of adult OCD sufferers experienced symptoms from ages 5–10. More than 20 percent had them by ages 10 to 15, and more than 40 percent had them by ages 15 to 20. In all, approximately 2 percent of the general population of children and adolescents meet OCD criteria.

Posttraumatic Stress Disorder: There are 3 risk factors that have demonstrated the likelihood that children will develop posttraumatic stress disorder: (1) the severity of the traumatic event, (2) parental reaction to the traumatic event, and (3) physical proximity to the traumatic event. As a general rule, most studies that have examined the risk factors associated with PTSD emergence in children find that children and adolescents reporting experiences with severe trauma also reported the greatest levels of PTSD-related symptoms. The extent of family support as well as parental coping capacities also correlate with symptom development in pediatric populations. Children and adolescents with a supportive family structure that has less chaos and acrimony between parents have a less acute PTSD symptom profile. Those with a lesser proximity from the traumatic event also report less distress.

There are a number of factors that affect the occurrence and severity of PTSD in youth. Interpersonal traumatic events such as rape and direct physical assault are more likely to result in PTSD as opposed to witnessing a school shooting or experiencing a natural or man-made disaster. Gender specific studies tell us that girls are more likely than boys to develop PTSD. Finally, it is not yet clear in what way a child's age at the time of the traumatic event exposure influences the occurrence or severity of PTSD. While some studies allude to a correlation, others simply do not.

Medication Management of Pediatric Anxiety Disorders

Studies on the medication management of anxiety disorders in youth are sparse and inconclusive, and there are few specific treatment guidelines. While benzodiazepines are used to treat anxiety and sleeplessness in children, the data supporting their use is minimal. While some anecdotal evidence has suggested possible benefit from Buspar (buspirone) in children, this remains a gray area. Antihistamines such as Benadryl (diphenhydramine) and Vistaril (hydroxyzine) have been used for decades to ameliorate anxiety symptoms in psychiatrically disturbed children. Anafranil (clomipramine), Luvox (fluvoxamine) and Zoloft (sertraline) have FDA- approved indications for children and adolescents with OCD. Experience with the SSRIs in controlled pediatric studies has led clinicians to consider these agents for treating non-OCD anxiety disorders as well. Controlled studies and supportive data are significantly lacking in the treatment of pediatric anxiety disorders with beta blockers.

Cognitive-behavioral interventions have proven to be effective for a majority of children and adolescents with anxiety disorders. Between 50 and 80 percent of children respond to well designed and effectively employed CBT treatment models, and at the completion of treatment no longer meet diagnostic criteria for the presenting anxiety disorder.

Psychotic Disorders

Psychotic disorders can involve an extreme impairment in the ability to distinguish reality from fantasy, behave in an emotionally appropriate manner, and communicate effectively. The National Institute of Health (NIH) indicates that schizophrenia is rare in children. Adolescent onset generally occurs between the ages of 11 and 15. Young people with schizophrenia have psychotic periods that can involve hallucinations, social isolation, poor reality testing, anhedonia (inability to experience pleasure) and delusional thoughts.

Medication Management of Child and Adolescent Psychotic Disorders

The preferred drugs in the treatment of psychotic disorders in children and adolescents are the atypical antipsychotics. Risperdal (risperidone), Abilify (aripiprazole), Zyprexa (olanzapine) and Seroquel (quetiapine) are FDA approved for the treatment of schizophrenia and bipolar disorder in adolescents and children.

As discussed in the section on childhood bipolar disorder, benefit-vs. - risk factors associated with the use of these drugs in youth are of considerable concern. With the approval of Zyprexa (olanzapine) and Seroquel (quetiapine), the FDA stated that it wants to know more about the risk of weight gain and diabetes in young people taking these medications and other antipsychotics as well. It has been clear for years that weight gain and other endocrine risks are associated with these medications and their warning labels indicate this. Evidence now suggests that these issues are even more paramount in youth.

CHAPTER 15

Attention Deficit Hyperactivity Disorder

As of this writing, The Centers for Disease Control (CDC) reports that nearly 20 percent of high school age boys in the U.S. and 11 percent of school-age children overall have received a diagnosis of ADHD. There's been a 53 percent rise in diagnosis in those ages 4–17 in this past decade alone. Two-thirds of those with a current diagnosis receive prescription stimulants. And even more adolescents will likely be prescribed medication because the American Psychiatric Association has changed the new onset diagnostic age requirement such that symptoms can appear before age 12 rather than before age 7, at it has been for years.

Given the statistics cited above, it is becoming increasingly evident that some prescribers are viewing even minor symptoms of distraction or inattentiveness worthy of an ADHD diagnosis. At the same time, pharmaceutical companies are crafting advertisements showcasing how medication can substantially improve a child's life. Such ads play to parents' fears by showing children struggling in school or abandoned by peers. Moreover, many parents are pressuring prescribers to prescribe drugs for the ailing child to make their lives easier. Here's a case example from a few months ago to illustrate:

Nine-year-old Megan's mother called my office. The purpose of her call was to set up a consultation whereby I would offer medication options for Megan's "ADHD." I wasn't asked to assess the child for ADHD—Julie, Megan's mother, merely wanted to discuss the range of drug options and which one(s) would be most suitable for her daughter.

We set up an appointment. Megan arrived in her school uniform accompanied by Julie. The crux of the presenting problem according to Julie is that Megan is routinely falling asleep each evening when instead she should be actively engaged in her homework. Julie went on to say that Megan's last evaluation report indicated that she had two C grades—not her customary straight A and occasional B performance. And because Megan's grades had fallen off, her homeroom teacher thought the child should be placed on medication to "help her focus."

I asked to see Megan for a few minutes alone. Julie refused, saying that Megan wouldn't offer up all of the "facts" and that I should just tell her what medications are best. I refused to do that stating that if any recommendations from me were to be forthcoming, I'd want to assess the situation first.

So Megan and I met and here's what I found out—information by the way, that was not volunteered by Julie. Three days per week, Julie picks Megan up from school and transports her to a gymnastics class, then to piano lessons and then to cheerleading practice back at school, all on the same afternoon. The little girl has no interest in gymnastics and cheerleading but loves learning to play the piano. Megan told me, "Mr. Joe, I fall asleep doing my homework because I'm tired. Would you please tell my mother this is too much?"

I did just that. Julie was unaccepting of this and told Megan to come along because they were leaving. I made one more try at explaining the dynamics of Megan's situation and why I believed she wasn't completing her homework. Julie refused to listen and away they went. There was no further contact between us.

Megan no more has ADHD than I do. Some children are increasingly being robbed of their childhood by those who are supposed to love them most. Some children's lives are over-scheduled and sometimes insanely stressful. They've barely learned their ABC's before they're diagnosed with ADHD.

Then there's the issue of some teachers acting as trained behavioral clinicians and indiscriminately recommending medication to potentially make their lives in the classroom easier—all at the expense of a child for whom there is no clear rationale for medication use in the first place.

Psychostimulants prescribed to children who meet the right symptom set can make a world of positive difference. This is where the focus should be—making life a bit less hard for affected children and adolescents.

OTHER ADHD CHARACTERISTICS

- Boys are 2–3 times more likely to develop ADHD than girls
- Observable in children as young as age 4; usual onset is age 7 to 8
- Often misdiagnosed due to its frequent co-occurrence with bipolar disorder, anxiety, depression, intellectual disability, borderline personality disorder, conduct disorder, oppositional defiant disorder, Tourette's syndrome and trauma experiences

- Accompanied by poor frustration tolerance, transitional difficulties, possible sleep disturbances and poor self-image

Adult ADHD

In the past few years, adult attention deficit hyperactivity disorder has garnered increasing attention. For years, conventional wisdom in the mental health field considered ADHD as a disorder of childhood and adolescence and believed that advancing age was accompanied by symptom remission. It's true that hyperactivity and impulsivity symptoms do abate for many adults diagnosed with ADHD in their youth, but it's also apparent that the core symptoms of distractibility and inattentiveness persist well into adulthood. Also, many if not most adults with attentional deficits were never diagnosed as children or adolescents. For adults with ADD, the responsibilities of keeping a job, paying bills and raising children can be quite problematic. Distractibility symptoms can make driving an automobile quite challenging. Marital problems can ensue as a result of poor listening skills and an inability to honor commitments. Adults with ADD are more likely to be restless and have difficulty relaxing as opposed to the classic hyperactivity symptoms exhibited by children. And procrastination, chronic tardiness, angry outbursts and failing to prioritize are common. Thus it is very important that these problematic issues be treated in adults with ADD. All of the medication classes used to treat children and adolescents discussed below can be employed in adults.

Mental distractibility is the core symptom of ADHD. Inattentiveness is characterized by difficulty paying attention for sustained periods; poor listening skills; losing needed items; carelessness; forgetfulness; difficulty organizing activities; failure to follow through on tasks; and avoiding activities that require prolonged mental effort.

The core features of hyperactivity and impulsivity are characterized by fidgeting or squirming; leaving one's seat during class; restlessness, running and climbing excessively; talking too much; responding to questions before the question is stated; interrupting others; and experiencing difficulty waiting for one's turn.

DSM-5 Changes to ADHD

ADHD's description and criteria have been repositioned and can be found in the Chapter on Neurodevelopmental Disorders. Also, the subtypes that have long defined the symptomatic presentation have been replaced with presentation specifiers. Here are three instances whereby a child can now meet criteria for an ADHD diagnosis: First, the child has inattention only; this is considered ADHD due to inattentiveness. Second, the child possesses hyperactivity and impulsivity characteristics; this is considered ADHD due to hyperactivity and impulsivity. Third, the child displays all three dimensions; this is referred to as the combined type.

ADHD ETIOLOGY

Though initial theories focused on ADHD as a disorder of hyperarousal, a different view of the disorder has emerged from rigorous clinical investigations. The current clinical thinking is that ADHD is a disorder of executive function accompanied by weakened "new brain" or prefrontal cortex circuitry that regulates attention and behavior. There is a significant genetic component associated with the disorder. As a result, norepinephrine and dopamine pathways are adversely affected. Both these neurotransmitters play a key role in the therapeutic effects of stimulant medications. Other theories focus on vitamin deficiencies, food additives and food allergies. Some nutritional approaches lean toward low-gluten diets and the addition of omega-3 fatty acid supplements. It is believed that ADHD does not develop from sugar consumption but that consuming sugary food groups may exacerbate symptoms.

THE MEDICATION EVALUATION

Obtaining an accurate history is absolutely essential to isolating ADHD as a diagnosis because co-occurring disorders are the rule rather than the exception when it comes to assessing mental syndromes in youth, and every mental disorder on the planet adversely affects attention in some manner regardless of age. Begin by asking questions about the individual's present "occupation." If the individual is a student, inquire about what sort of difficulties he or she may be having in school, particularly at the university or college level when the rigors of assimilating and accommodating information, studying and test-taking tend to peak. Ask those in the work force how they're doing on the job and whether they've moved from job to job over a short time period. You want to be sure not to overlook benign signs that may indicate ADHD, such as the person getting lost on the way to your office, difficulty filling out office paperwork, frequent loss of items such as keys, cellphones and the like, and routinely failing to complete tasks such as reading a book in its entirety. And then there is the family tree, so be sure to inquire about whether the individual's siblings or parents have possibly been diagnosed with ADHD.

MEDICATION TREATMENTS FOR ADHD

There are three classes of medications with proven effectiveness in the treatment of ADHD: psychostimulants, some antidepressants, and alpha 2 adrenergic agonists.

Medications for ADHD	
Brand Name	Generic Name
Adderall	dextroamphetamine/amphetamine
Adderall XR	dextroamphetamine/amphetamine
Concerta	methylphenidate
Daytrana	methylphenidate transdermal
Dexedrine	dextroamphetamine
Dexedrine Spansule	dextroamphetamine
Dextrostat	dextroamphetamine
Focalin	dexmethylphenidate
Focalin XR	dexmethylphenidate
Intuniv	guanfacine ER
Metadate CD	methylphenidate
Methylin	methylphenidate
Quillivant XR	methylphenidate liquid
Ritalin	methylphenidate
Ritalin LA, SR	methylphenidate
Strattera	atomoxetine
Tenex	guanfacine
Vyvanse	lisdexamfetamine
Wellbutrin	bupropion
Wellbutrin SR, XL	bupropion sustained release

Psychostimulants

The treatment of ADHD with psychostimulants has undergone a long but steady evolutionary process over the last five decades. All of the psychostimulants, regardless of their onset of action or duration of action, increase prefrontal cortex levels of norepinephrine and dopamine. As a result, the attentional deficits and behavioral manifestations associated with ADHD generally improve.

The first stimulants employed were immediate-release preparations of Ritalin (methylphenidate), Dexedrine (dextroamphetamine) followed by the mixed amphetamine salt Adderall. A typical dosing regimen with these medications is to administer them three times daily—often at 8 a.m., noon and 4 p.m. At issue with the immediate-release preparations is that symptoms may return between doses, resulting in an unstable clinical course, so a child's school performance could typically worsen until the next dose is administered. Also, a multiple daily dosing regimen is inconvenient, and this fosters noncompliance. However, immediate release preparations offer greater dosing flexibility and often are less expensive.

The standard of care for treating ADHD now includes longer acting, once-daily preparations. An example of the newer generation, long-acting methylphenidate drugs is Concerta (methylphenidate). Concerta (methylphenidate) was designed to provide 12 hours of symptom coverage by essentially replacing three doses of immediate-release methylphenidate administered four hours apart. This 12-hour symptom management recognizes the importance of covering the school day and after-school hours, including homework. Debate abounds as to whether the 12-hour coverage claim for Concerta (methylphenidate) is accurate. Many users and prescribers report symptom management to be closer to 7–8 hours.

Concerta was then followed by other methylphenidate preparations, such as Metadate CD and Ritalin LA—both of which are methylphenidate extended-release preparations. Also, an extended release mixed amphetamine salts (MAS-XR) product, Adderall XR, is widely prescribed.

Daytrana (methylphenidate transdermal system) is a transdermal methylphenidate patch that is absorbed through the skin, thereby bypassing some metabolism through the liver. The patch is typically worn for up to 9 hours and offers flexibility in that the duration of delivery can be customized. If children have a short school day they can remove the patch earlier; if they have a longer day—including homework that extends into the evening hours— they can continue wearing the patch. Initially it was thought that Daytrana (methylphenidate transdermal system) would have fewer side effects compared to oral methylphenidate, but this does not seem to be true. Also, because the patch strength doesn't exceed 30mg, dosing problems emerge, with users often having to wear multiple patches at the same time.

Vyvanse (lisdexamfetamine dimesylate) is yet another long-acting agent to control ADHD symptoms throughout the day. It is rapidly absorbed from the gastrointestinal tract and converted to dextroamphetamine and the amino acid l-lysine. The therapeutic action of Vyvanse (lisdexamfetamine dimesylate) is not realized unless the drug is swallowed and then completely absorbed by the gastrointestinal tract. This means it may possess lower abuse potential via intranasal and intravenous routes of administration when compared with other oral psychostimulants. Vyvanse (lisdexamphetamine dimesylate) is not very long-acting; some users claim it provides no more than 6–7 hours of symptom coverage.

Quillivant XR (methylphenidate ER suspension) establishes itself as the first, once-daily, extended-release formulation of liquid methylphenidate for ADHD. In simple terms this is a long-acting liquid Ritalin (methylphenidate). There are a number of people who have trouble swallowing pills and capsules. This formulation will be particularly helpful to younger children who fear swallowing solid preparations and elderly individuals with swallowing difficulties. This drug will also be useful for those in need of dosage "fine tuning."

Quillivant XR (methylphenidate ER suspension) doesn't involve the opening of capsules and sprinkling the contents on food or placing it in other liquids, thus making dosage titration much easier and streamlined.

Quillivant XR's (methylphenidate ER suspension) delivery system is exactly the same as with other XR products such as Concerta (methylphenidate). The active ingredient is "pulsed" into the bloodstream at select intervals throughout the day, providing eight hour symptom coverage.

Long-term use of psychostimulants is generally well tolerated. Common side effects include insomnia (particularly at the beginning of treatment), dry mouth, decrease in appetite and weight loss, minor changes in heart rate and blood pressure, and a rebound effect whereby symptoms can worsen as the medication effects wear off. Weight loss is transient; most young subjects catch up in weight as well as height throughout the developmental cycle. There is some evidence that stimulants suppress the secretion of growth hormone during the years these medications are typically administered. Prescribers often gradually introduce dose reductions as patients get older, and at ages 14 to 16, most children have a growth spike regardless of medication use. Psychostimulants are considered C-II controlled substances by the FDA.

Antidepressants

Wellbutrin (bupropion) and Wellbutrin SR (bupropion sustained-release) can be helpful in treating ADHD, because like the psychostimulants, they can enhance the actions of norepinephrine and dopamine in the prefrontal cortex. SSRIs on the other hand, due to their singular effects on serotonin, are considered poor choices in managing ADHD. From an efficacy perspective, clinical trials indicate a clear advantage of stimulant use over Wellbutrin (bupropion). However Wellbutrin (bupropion), as an antidepressant, can treat co-occurring depression and is not a controlled substance.

Strattera (atomoxetine) is a norepinephrine specific reuptake inhibitor (NRI) antidepressant. It carries the same "black box" warning as do all other antidepressants for possible risk of suicide when used by children and adolescents. It was first marketed for adult ADHD before gaining FDA approval for use in children. Strattera (atomoxetine) fails miserably in head-to-head clinical trials versus the psychostimulants in managing ADHD, and long-term safety data on Strattera (atomoxetine) for use in children is not well established. Strattera (atmoxetine) has been linked to liver damage.

Alpha-2 Agonists

Tenex (guanfacine) is an antihypertensive used to control high blood pressure. It can also be utilized to treat some anxiety conditions and to control hyperactivity, aggression, irritability, tics and Tourette's syndrome. It can be combined with the psychostimulants discussed above. Tenex (guanfacine) acts directly on the prefrontal cortex to improve the so-called "executive functions," including organization, planning and foresight. In September 2009, the FDA gave its blessing to a long-acting formulation of guanfacine—Intuniv (guanfacine ER). Intuniv (guanfacine ER) is approved for the treatment of ADHD in children and adolescents ages 6–17. Intuniv (guanfacine ER) dosing is not well established in adults. Side effects of Tenex (guanfacine) and Intuniv (guanfacine ER) are generally mild. They include possible dizziness from low blood pressure, headache, nausea, drowsiness and slight changes in heart rhythm.

DRUG HOLIDAYS

The issue of drug holidays—short-term, deliberate discontinuation of medication—is also known as a structured treatment interruption. These "holidays" can take place over a weekend, a full week or an extended school vacation. There is no definitive conclusion regarding the benefits or risks of drug holidays. Some prescribers maintain that because ADHD is a chronic disorder, suspending treatment is not in the patient's best interest. But for parents who are concerned about "over drugging" their children, drug holidays can be a welcome relief, even if only a perceived one.

According to a 2005 report in *Medscape Psychiatry and Mental Health*, there are three reasons for a drug holiday:

- To demonstrate the clinical need for medication
- To provide a break from side effects

- To satisfy the notion of caregivers that medication should not be used if it can be avoided.

Weekend holidays from psychostimulants can minimize insomnia and appetite loss without significantly increasing ADHD symptoms, however anecdotal reports by some physicians indicate that patients can experience difficulty readjusting to regular dosing after the drug holiday is completed.

OTHER INTERVENTIONS FOR MANAGING ADHD

Youth with ADHD are immersed in an ongoing struggle to keep their lives manageable. They are prone to general messiness and disorganization in the major areas of their lives—home, school and social situations. They routinely lose homework assignments and fail to complete them. An exhaustive review of structural, behavioral and organizational interventions is beyond the scope of this book, so here are a few simple recommendations to bring some measure of order and structure to their lives and help them succeed:

- For easily distracted children with ADHD, simplify their living and study environment by clearing clutter to help them focus better. Engage them in the clean-up process and enlist their help with organizing, labeling and getting the important things they need properly placed.
- Create to-do lists, important reminders and schedules. Get the whole family involved and make it a fun project by scheduling an outing to a local hobby shop to purchase colored pens, poster board and lists with cute sayings or clever illustrations.
- Post a large family calendar in an area of the home where family members most often congregate. Make it the child's responsibility to enter important events, dates and appointments on the calendar.
- Establish routines for key periods during the day (morning, bedtime), homework and other outside or social activities. For each routine, make a list of what needs to be completed and in what time frame. Then try it out and change up the order of the list until it's most manageable and can be efficiently executed.

For Parents and Caretakers

Consider the possibility of ADHD in your child if:

- It is obvious that in multiple milieus (school, play, home) it seems impossible for your child to sit and focus without becoming easily distracted and inattentive within even just a few minutes.

- The child has much difficulty following directions and playing by the rules—for example, when "quiet time" is required.

- The child is being shunned and possibly is being treated like a pariah by teachers, peers and even family members because he or she is so difficult to be around.

- The child has never done well academically and is consistently failing.

- The child is spending an inordinate amount of time in "time-outs" (mostly for younger kids) or in some type of "punish hall" for older children.

- The child is not responding to multiple attempts at redirection.

- The child's distractibility and impulse control problems *aren't* leading to marked maliciousness, meanness, or attempts to perpetrate harm on others. If these issues are present, it's likely something else, not ADHD.

- A trial of stimulants has resulted in objective, measurable positive changes in ability to focus and behave more appropriately without excessive movement.

Dosage Range Chart—Medications for ADD/ADHD		
Brand Name	**Generic Name**	**Daily Dosage Range***
Adderall	dextroamphetamine/ amphetamine	5mg – 40mg
Adderall XR	dextroamphetamine/ amphetamine extended release	10mg – 30mg
Concerta	methylphenidate	18mg – 108mg
Daytrana	methylphenidate	10mg – 30mg (transdermal)
Dexedrine	dextroamphetamine	5mg – 40mg
Focalin	dexmethylphenidate	5mg – 40 mg
Focalin XR	dexmethylphenidate	10mg – 40mg
Intuniv	guanfacine ER	1mg – 4mg
Metadate CD	methylphenidate	20mg – 60mg
Methylin	methylphenidate	10mg – 60 mg
Quillivant XR	methylphenidate liquid	20mg – 60mg
Ritalin	methylphenidate	5mg – 50mg
Ritalin LA	methylphenidate	20mg – 40mg
Strattera	atomoxetine	60mg – 120mg
Tenex	guanfacine	0.25mg – 1.0mg **
Vyvanse	lisdexamfetamine	30mg – 70mg
Wellbutrin SR, XL	bupropion	150mg – 300mg
(sustained release)		
* Suggested adult dose		
** Dosed 2 to 3 times daily		
Note: Dosage ranges may vary depending on source, and may also vary according to age.		

CHAPTER 16

Herbals and Supplements

To read the volumes of ever-increasing information on this subject, the latest "natural" miracle cure is either on the horizon or already here. There are many claims to fame in that regard, but most of them fall by the wayside if and when they are subjected to scientific research. You have no doubt seen in your practice the increased use of "self- prescribed" alternative remedies, often utilized by patients regardless of whether these remedies were recommended by their health practitioners. For this reason, I am including these alternatives. My goal is to help you become aware of their uses, recommended dosages, side effects and possibly adverse actions.

Of the literally hundreds of herbals, supplements and vitamins that are touted as being effective, five have emerged with various levels of documented efficacy in the treatment of mental health disorders. This is by no means a complete list, and many experts disagree on the definitions of efficacy, but these are the ones that demonstrate credible evidence to back up their claims.

However, simply because they are not prescription drugs does not mean they don't have side effects, which, like those of any medication, can range from unpleasant to dangerous. It is therefore important for clinicians to know whether patients are taking any of the following, or any other alternative treatments for their conditions. Clinicians must then monitor for interactions and possible adverse effects.

St. John's Wort

This yellow wildflower, named after St. John the Baptist, became an "overnight sensation" in America after being used for thousands of years in Europe, and even by Native Americans, for a variety of ailments. It has risen to the top as probably one of the most effective herbal remedies in the treatment of mild depression. Once thought to mimic the actions of the monoamine oxidase inhibitors (MAOIs), recent findings indicate that it is more likely

Possible Side Effects of Alternative Remedies

ST. JOHN'S WORT

Restlessness, fatigue, dizziness and increased sensitivity to sunlight (photosensitivity).

May interact with oral contraceptives and reduce their effectiveness. Potentially serious interactions with prescription antidepressants, resulting in rapid heartbeat, agitation, tremors and other symptoms of elevated serotonin levels in the brain (serotonin syndrome).

SAM-e

Gastrointestinal symptoms (stomach upset, nausea, vomiting), insomnia, anxiety. May interact with some prescription antidepressants, resulting in rapid heartbeat, agitation, tremors and other symptoms of elevated serotonin levels in the brain (serotonin syndrome).

Warning: SAMe should not be used in patients with bipolar disorder (manic-depressive illness).

MELATONIN

Gastrointestinal symptoms, drowsiness, depression, headache, lethargy, ovulation inhibition and suppression of male sex drive. Risk of additional sedation if combined with alcohol. May interfere with corticosteroids such as prednisone.

GINKGO BILOBA

Headache, dizziness, restlessness, racing heart and gastrointestinal symptoms.

Caution should be exercised in patients with diabetes, hypoglycemia or other blood-sugar issues as ginkgo biloba can theoretically affect blood sugar levels. Monitoring is recommended for patients taking other medications that affect blood sugar.

Can affect the outcome of electroconvulsive therapy (ECT).

OMEGA-3 FATTY ACIDS

Increased risk of bruising.

May increase the risk of bleeding when combined with aspirin or other blood thinners.

VITAMIN D

Most people do not experience side effects with vitamin D unless too much is taken.

Some side effects of excessive vitamin D intake include weakness, sleepiness, fatigue, headache, dry mouth and nausea.

---

similar in action to the SSRIs, leading to its nickname of "Nature's Prozac." One area of similarity to the MAOIs, however, is the high incidence of drug/drug interactions that occur with St. John's Wort. For this reason, this herbal is almost always recommended to be taken alone. This minimizes, as much as possible, the significant and potentially problematic interactions with prescription medications or other herbals. Complicating matters further, St. John's Wort is not a single substance. Rather, it is a complex mix of at least 10 groups of active ingredients that involve antidepressant, anti-inflammatory, antibacterial, antiviral, sedative and diuretic properties.

One of the problems with determining drug interactions associated with St. John's Wort is that, as an herbal, it is not FDA-regulated. Because of its pharmacology, St. John's Wort should not be used in combination with prescription serotonin reuptake inhibitors. This combination can lead to serotonin syndrome with its symptoms of mania, hypomania, anxiety, agitation, rigidity and fever. Also, St. John's Wort should be avoided by pregnant women. Studies show that this herbal can reduce the anticoagulant effect of the blood thinner warfarin and can lower plasma concentrations of the cardiac medication digoxin. It is also known to decrease the efficacy of oral contraceptives. One side effect of St. John's Wort is photosensitivity, or an abnormal sensitivity to light, especially of the eyes.

St. John's Wort has been used extensively in Germany, where many of the most notable studies have taken place. Although this herbal has been successful in treating mild to moderate depression—enough to earn approval from Germany's Commission E—its effects on major depressive disorder are less promising. The usual adult dose is 900 mg per day, usually in divided doses of 300 mg each.

SAMe (S-ADENOSYLMETHIONINE)

SAMe is considered by many to be one of the best natural antidepressants in the treatment of mild to moderate depression. This made SAMe headline news when it first hit the U.S. market in 1999. SAMe is a substance found in the body that helps in the production of neurotransmitters and hormones aided by the amino acid methionine. Ordinarily, the brain manufactures all the SAMe it needs, but in depression, methionine synthesis is impaired.

SAMe has been the subject of more than 100 trials around the world. Some of these studies show that it effectively mimics the action of the selective serotonin reuptake inhibitors (SSRIs), which we have previously discussed as instrumental in the treatment of depression. In some recent studies, SAMe has performed as well as antidepressant drugs, including SSRIs. It is also used in the treatment of fibromyalgia, a chronic disorder characterized by widespread muscle pain accompanied by depression and anxiety. Although there is no standard dose, SAMe appears to be effective particularly in mild depression at doses of 400 mg per day.

In 2004 researchers from Harvard Medical School found that SAMe was beneficial in treatment-resistant depression by combining it with conventional antidepressants for those whose symptoms had not responded to the antidepressant alone. The results of this study showed a positive response to the therapy, with improved scores on the Hamilton Depression Scale and Montgomery-Asberg Depression Rating scale, two instruments that measure the severity of depression.

A 1994 report of 13 clinical trials concluded that the efficacy of SAMe in treating depressive syndromes and disorders is superior to that of placebo and comparable to that of standard tricyclic antidepressants. These findings were confirmed in a 2002 report presented by the Agency for Healthcare Research and Quality.

Due to its high cost, SAMe has never really taken off as a treatment for depression in the United States. A one-month supply in its oral form can run as high as $60, putting SAMe in line, cost-wise, with some prescription antidepressants. Also, people with bipolar disorder should not take SAMe due to a number of reported cases whereby patients have experienced manic or hypomanic episodes.

MELATONIN

Melatonin can be your best friend if you have difficulty getting to sleep. It is a hormone manufactured by the pineal gland in the brain from the amino acid tryptophan. Melatonin may be connected to letting our bodies know when it is time to fall sleep and wake up. Melatonin is synthesized and released during darkness, and natural levels are present in the blood prior to bedtime. In people older than 40 years, the pineal gland has likely slowed down its production of melatonin, and by age 50, virtually everyone has a melatonin deficiency. Melatonin is primarily used in cases of insomnia, and it may also be taken to prevent jet lag associated with long air travel.

According to the NIMH, multiple human studies have measured the effects of melatonin supplements on sleep in healthy individuals. Although most of the trials have been small and brief, the weight of scientific evidence suggests that melatonin decreases the time needed to fall asleep, increases feelings of sleepiness, and increases the duration of sleep. For use in adults in the management of insomnia, doses within the range of 0.6mg—3mg at bedtime, preferably one hour before retiring, are generally sufficient.

There is also some suggestion that melatonin can improve sleep disorders associated with Alzheimer's disease, specifically night time agitation and poor sleep quality, but further research is needed. In addition, a limited study of patients with bipolar disorder attempted to determine if insomnia or irregular sleep patterns could be improved with melatonin, but no clear benefits were reported.

Another area of melatonin research by the NIMH addressed sleep disturbances in children with neuro-psychiatric disorders, such as mental retardation, autism and psychiatric disorders. These studies demonstrated a reduced time to fall asleep, an increased duration of sleep, and credible scientific evidence for its use.

Areas in which further study of melatonin is required include ADHD in children, benzodiazepine tapering, sleep disturbances associated with depression and schizophrenia, and the use of melatonin to treat tardive dyskinesia.

GINKGO BILOBA

Ginkgo biloba is one of the top-selling herbal supplements in the United States. With an aging population and the attendant scare of Alzheimer's disease, people have been buying ginkgo for years in the hopes that it will improve their memory. Since the 1950s, more than 400 papers on ginkgo biloba—the majority from German investigators—have appeared in the medical literature. Unfortunately, ginkgo biloba has failed in trials with regard to memory improvement. But there is good news: The scientific literature suggests that ginkgo biloba benefits those with early-stage Alzheimer's and multi-infarct dementia (memory loss due to disruption in blood flow to the brain). In fact, ginkgo biloba may actually be as helpful as the Alzheimer's drug Aricept (donepezil), in that it appears to slow cognitive decline in dementia.

A report published by the Oregon Health Sciences University and the Portland Veterans Affairs Medical Center synthesized the data from four major controlled studies. They show that there was a "small but significant effect" from treatment of three to six months with 120 mg to 140 mg of ginkgo biloba extract on objective measures of cognitive function in Alzheimer's.

Ginkgo biloba appears to work most effectively in disorders having to do with circulatory problems, both neurodegenerative and vascular diseases that involve poor blood flow to the brain due to narrowed blood vessels or strokes. It is a potent antioxidant (that is, it protects cells from damage), and its main agents are thought to be unique chemicals called ginkgolides. It is also an anticoagulant—meaning it reduces the stickiness of blood platelets and the formation of blood clots—and has anti-inflammatory properties.

Traditional Chinese Medicine (TCM) practitioners have for thousands of years used ginkgo biloba derived from a tree native to China and Japan. Extracts of this herbal have been used to treat a variety of disorders. So far it is showing its best results—in addition to slowing cognitive decline—in the management of intermittent claudication, which is leg pain due to insufficient circulation; and cerebral insufficiency, a syndrome secondary to atherosclerotic disease characterized by confusion, impaired concentration, dizziness, anxiety and depression. Ginkgo biloba may also help improve blood flow to the heart, provide an immune system boost, and help to reduce free radical damage.

OMEGA-3 FATTY ACIDS

A particular type of fat is so essential, that our body cells can literally collapse without it. Fish oil—with its singular component omega-3 fatty acids in conjunction with other types of fat in the membranes that surround the cells—literally control cell behavior.

Fish oils are made up of EPA (eicosapentaenoic acid), critical in heart function, and DHA (docosahexaenoic acid), critical in brain function. These oils are found in fatty fish like salmon, mackerel, tuna and sardines, as well as in supplements in gel cap form. Both DHA and EPA affect calcium, sodium, and potassium ion channels that regulate cellular electrical activity in the heart and the brain.

Omega-3 fatty acids have been well established with regard to improving nerve conduction, and they are well on their way to being recognized as effective in the management of depression by regulating neurotransmitters like serotonin and dopamine. Studies have shown a correlation between low levels of omega-3s and depression, and trials using omega-3s are showing promising results in the use of this supplement as a treatment for depression. For example, a 2002 study was conducted in England with 60 men and women suffering from treatment-resistant depression (depression that did not respond to conventional medications). Those taking 1 gram of EPA per day showed significantly greater improvement on depression- measuring scales than did the placebo group.

In another study, this one of 30 patients with bipolar disorder led by a researcher at Harvard Medical School, the group that took 9.6 grams of omega-3 acids daily (EPA and DHA) showed "significant symptom reduction and a better outcome when compared to placebo [olive oil alone]." The conclusion was that the omega-3 fatty acids were well tolerated and improved the short-term course of illness.

The typical American diet is high in omega-6 compared to omega-3, prompting experts to recommend at least three servings of fish a week to maintain a balance between omega-3 and omega-6 fatty acids. While omega-6 oils (corn, soybean) can generate an inflammatory reaction, omega-3 oils found in cold-water fish work by subduing inflammation, which is why they are often used to alleviate the symptoms of rheumatoid arthritis, cancer, and Crohn's disease. The human body can also manufacture omega-3s from walnuts and flaxseed.

According to some experts, the rising rates of depression in this country could be partially explained by the rising ratios in omega-6 fatty acids. Although there is no conclusive proof of this theory, some practitioners are recommending "mood enhancing diets" for their patients that include eating more fish and adding an omega-3 supplement. In Japan and other countries where fish consumption is high, the rates of depression and heart disease are comparatively low.

Vitamin D

Vitamin D is produced in the body when the body is exposed to sunlight. Often referred to as the "sunshine" vitamin, levels can become depleted during the late fall and extending into the winter months when people tend to stay inside for longer periods of time and sunlight is less intense. A recent study in the *New England Journal of Medicine*, and a few others, indicated that low vitamin D levels correlate with depression. Nevertheless, two key questions linger: Do low vitamin D levels influence depression? Or does depression influence low vitamin D levels? These questions will remain unanswered until more numerous and larger full-scale studies which address causation are conducted.

CHAPTER 17

Solving Medication Challenges

Working with clients who need psychotropic medications presents several unique and thorny challenges. For example, how should you deal with clients who refuse, for various reasons, to take their medications? How best to work with well-meaning but poorly informed family members? When does "just enough" medication spill over into "too much?" How best to improve your relationships with physicians? Here is advice on how to meet these and other medication challenges.

HELPING CLIENTS OVERCOME RESISTANCE TO PSYCHOTROPIC MEDICATION

Why are some clients so resistant to the use of psychotropic medication? After all, medication intervention is a treatment strategy that has garnered widespread acceptance as an option for treating a vast array of mental health maladies.

Here are four common reasons why clients refuse or even downright resist medication, together with strategies you can use to help them better comprehend why medication might be a viable alternative for their condition:

1. The Shame Factor. Shame is often experienced as the voice in a client's head that judges what they do as wrong, inferior or somehow worthless. Clearly, these shaming inner voices can do considerable damage to clients' self-esteem. For some clients, this critical judge provides a continuously negative evaluation of what they are doing, moment-by-moment. If medication is mentioned as a treatment option, negative self-evaluation can kick into overdrive, resulting in faulty, illogical conclusions. Two common conclusions that clients reach are: (a) they have failed themselves because their own attempts to remedy their condition haven't worked, and (b) they must therefore be "really sick."

How you can help: First, work with the client on the negative self-talk. Emphasize that the resolution of their presenting problem is a journey that may include several directional paths, and that medication is merely one of these paths. Explain that medications are not necessarily essential, not demeaning or even redemptive. Medications are merely an option to help kick-start symptom improvement, an option that can be discontinued—preferably after consultation with their therapist and prescriber—if the client so wishes.

2. Family Interference. Face it, family members are our de-facto healthcare specialists. They have likely witnessed the unpredictability and even the anguish associated with the mental health struggles of their ill family member—your client. In this sense, they are not merely uninvolved bystanders. So for clinicians who want to practice in a context of collaborative care, expanding the scope of treatment to include family members is a must. Clients who believe their family has a supportive interest in their improvement are often less resistant to the use of psychotropic medication. Unfortunately, some family members, because of belief systems ingrained over many years, actually condone resistance to medication use, setting up a potential treatment challenge.

    How you can help: While maintaining a healthy respect for family members' views and experiences about medication, do challenge with determination their faulty belief systems—such as "mental illness is a character flaw," "medication is for crazy people," and "medication doesn't work." Provide family members with as much information as possible, including reading material and Web addresses. Answer their questions straightforwardly, as you will need them as allies in the treatment process.

3. Ambivalence. Practitioners at all levels of experience know that getting clients to overcome their resistance toward psychotropic medication is not necessarily easy. Many clients assess the odds associated with considering medication options for some time before making the commitment to pharmacotherapy as part of the treatment process. A client's decision therefore may be long and drawn out.

    How you can help: Patience is the key. Any attempt to rush the client into a premature decision is likely to backfire. It could also compromise the therapeutic relationship. Of course, waiting for clients to decide does not mean a clinician cannot offer an opinion. On the contrary, if the clinician knows that evidence-based literature supports a pharmacological treatment of a particular condition, then this information should be conveyed to the client. Again, offering reading material and reputable Web addresses can help ensure that clients have as much information as possible. Also, encourage them to ask questions, and then provide straightforward answers. This will help to demystify the decision-making process. In this way, the client can make informed choices regarding the importance of medication for their particular disorder.

4. Fear. Two often-expressed issues that invoke clients' fear of psychotropic medication are: (a) medication will, in some way, "change who they are," or alter their personality, and (b) although their troublesome symptoms may improve, intolerable side effects will be possibly worse than the illness itself.

> **How you can help:** It is imperative that a clinician stress that prescribed medications do <u>not</u> alter core personality, nor do they change someone into something they are not. Explain that medication does not change behavior, but has the capacity to ameliorate symptoms that are wreaking havoc in the client's life. Inform the client that all drugs have side effects, and that some of these side effects may indeed be of concern. For example, while lithium use is linked to possible coma and even death, such circumstances are very rare and most often associated with individuals that misuse this drug and don't comply with the required blood work. In the end, clients need to know that only <u>they can make the decision to get better.</u> So ask your client, "Are you willing to tolerate some weight gain as a trade-off for feeling better and becoming more functional?" Or: "If weight gain becomes a bothersome issue, would you commit to working on diet modification and a regular exercise regimen?"

One of the biggest challenges for clinicians is respecting a client's decision to resist medication use, even in the face of continuing, and sometimes debilitating, symptoms. There is a fine line between coercing vs. encouraging medication use, and the misuse of power in the clinical relationship can undermine client self-determination. Also, it's worth remembering that when it comes to medication, clients will make their own choices—on their own terms and in their own time.

THE INTERACTION BETWEEN FAMILIES AND PSYCHOTROPIC MEDICATION

Family members can have a significant influence on a client's initial decision to utilize psychotropic medication. Family members can also influence the client's willingness to adhere to a treatment regimen once it has been started. Most clients live in families, and they are affected by their loved ones' responses to their choices. For these reasons, clinicians should welcome input from members of the client's family. After all, the responsibility of caring for a client usually falls on family members; they are not simply uninvolved bystanders. For example, it is common for family members to prompt or even coerce a client into making the initial appointment with the clinician. However, due to the stigma of mental illness, and the client's concerns about being a burden to family members, the family may not be fully aware of the client's mental health status. This lack of knowledge often results from fractured relationships in the family and the client's preference to keep family members out of the loop.

Although only a few studies have examined the interaction between families and psychotropic medication, we can still extract some clinical wisdom from the sparse literature. It makes sense that caring families would be concerned about their ill family member and would therefore be affected by his or her behavior. But these studies tell us that while a collaborative approach to treatment—one that includes family members—works best, families are seldom consulted about medication or educated about the ill client's condition. Of similar concern is how little clinicians utilize family members as collateral sources of information about the ill client's previous history.

Why not? Well, family work is time-consuming, and clinicians are often hamstrung by clients who won't sign informed consent documents that would allow the family to participate in treatment. Also, family work can be cumbersome from the standpoint of scheduling appointments—getting them together can be as difficult as the proverbial herding of cats. What's more, time constraints, fueled by managed care-imposed restrictions on the number of sessions that clinicians can conduct with clients, makes it even easier to overlook family member input. There is also the <u>family's</u> belief system regarding medication to consider.

In spite of these obstacles, clinicians are encouraged to engage clients in permitting family to participate in treatment decision-making. Clients who believe their family members have a supportive interest in their improvement are often more willing to submit to a psychotropic medication evaluation. That's because caring families hope that medication—accompanied by other non-pharmacological, psychosocial treatment strategies—will ease their loved one's suffering. This can also improve relationships between the client and their family.

When getting the family on board, explain why you believe a psychotropic medication evaluation is worth considering for their loved one. Maintain a healthy respect for family members' views and experiences about medication, but do challenge faulty belief systems with determination. As you would with clients, also offer reading material and Web addresses to family members to ensure that they have as much information as possible. Also, be sure to answer their questions as straightforwardly as possible; when you invest in client success, you need all the allies you can get.

SIX TIPS FOR IMPROVED RELATIONSHIPS WITH PHYSICIANS AND OTHER PRESCRIBERS

Non-medical clinicians train and practice in a world that is considerably different from that of physicians and other medication prescribers. (Use of the word physician in this section includes other prescribers). With the employment of the medical model and the liberal use of psychotropic medications to alter faulty biochemistry, knowledge and appreciation of medical culture is more important than ever before in strengthening collaborative relationships with physicians.

Therapists at times are reluctant to collaborate with physicians who are intimidating, boorish, insulting, controlling or egotistical. Physicians also carry their own stereotypes of therapists as being too "theory oriented," "touchy-feely" or not "symptom focused." These contradicting viewpoints demand that professionals sharing client care become familiar with each other's role and respect the value of each other's views and opinions. For the non-medical clinician though, respect for the hierarchy is a key component in building relationships with doctors.

Here are six tips for proactively improving your interaction with physicians:

- Approach physicians in an assertive, confident manner. This will endear you to doctors faster than anything else. If you find yourself apprehensive or anxious, jot down your points or questions on an index card or notepad. Be succinct and make eye contact.

- If you work at an on-site system, find the "main traffic area" and place yourself in the middle of it. Greet physicians as they walk by with a smile and, where appropriate, a handshake. This builds good will with an ally you are going to need.

- Establish your expertise as a competent worker and respond in a timely way to physicians who reach out to you. Once you establish your competence, you will become the "go-to" person, particularly for difficult cases.

- Speak the "language." This means focusing on symptoms and eschewing any theory jargon. For example, if Ms. Jones reports feeling nauseous, restless and agitated after a few days on Cymbalta, convey these symptoms using these terms to the prescriber. This is not the time to discuss Ms. Jones' repressed memories from childhood!

- Never recommend a specific medication treatment. Unless the physician has specifically asked you for a suggestion, this is an egregious boundary violation. While the client system may give input, the final medication decision should be made by the physician.

- Understand and appreciate cultural differences. Physicians are under severe time constraints that need to be respected. Physicians take a tremendous amount of responsibility for their patients' well- being, and they facilitate change in their patients' conditions. Non- medical clinicians, on the other hand, often place responsibility for change on the backs of their patients. This difference of perspective can create a conflict between physicians and clinicians and skew their expectations of one another.

Here's the key: To work collaboratively with physicians, recognize and appreciate the ways in which their role differs from your own.

WHEN TO CHANGE DOCTORS

Most of us are conditioned to believe that our doctor or prescriber has our best interest in mind, and in the vast majority of instances this is true. But it's also true that some relationships—regardless of context—reach an impasse where consideration needs to be given to moving on—not finding fault. I've received hundreds of e-mails from folks who report what they believe to be a communications breakdown between themselves and their doctor. Another complaint I often receive is that treatment not only isn't yielding results but is contributing to the problem or situation actually getting worse. So if this is happening to you or one of your clients, here are some tips for when, metaphorically speaking, it might be time to pick up the bat and ball and head to another playing field:

1. **Appointment times are routinely ignored and the doctor is regularly running late.** Whether it's the doctor going overtime with a patient,

scheduling problems or an office in chaos, waiting in excess of 20–30 minutes beyond the scheduled appointment time is annoying and a sign that something is amiss. Sure, emergencies arise and stuff happens, but such situations should be the exception, not the rule.

2. **Basic questions pursuant to appropriate care are brushed off.** What do you think is wrong with me? What might be causing this? What else could it be? Such questions deserve cogent answers at some point in treatment. If not, it's like sailing on a rudderless ship with no destination in sight.

3. **The doctor is distracted, disengaged or is staring at a computer screen during a session.** Any patient should have their doctor's full attention during a visit. This is as basic as it gets. I'm hearing more and more from people that technology is interfering with their appointments.

4. **One medication after another is being prescribed to no avail and no other treatment direction is being discussed.** This perplexes and even angers patients when said strategy is not getting results, no clear rationale is offered and alternative modes of treatment aren't addressed. As a patient of mine commented last week, "I don't trust him anymore."

5. **When respectfully challenged, the response is curt, intended to show "who's the boss" or the patient is just ignored.** It's hard to maintain respect for anyone who does this, but when it comes from a professional that we typically hold in high esteem and from whom we don't expect such behavior, it's best to put the relationship in the rear view mirror.

The association that patients have with their doctors is typically a treasured one, but when trust erodes and respect is lost, it's not as much about who is at fault as it is about seeking out greener pastures.

THE 15-MINUTE MED CHECK

Or maybe … 20 minutes. This is the #1 issue, complaint-wise, that I hear from my clients when it comes to working with their psychiatrist. In this model, patients are like experimental subjects representative of their symptoms and complaints, and are objectified in such a way that treating their faulty brain chemistry or whatever else the medication is supposed to do for them is the primary goal. So unfortunately, there's little partnering with the patient in the 15-minute model and the meeting environment not only defines the parameters of the session, it establishes the doctor as the one who knows best—rendering this much like a drug trial with one subject. In traditional, well-designed drug trials, subjects are often seen weekly and are exposed to lots of contact with other professionals as well as support systems that include receiving psychotherapy.

It's a bit of a stretch to conclude that time constraints are a valid reason for not seeking the patient's point of view and treatment preferences. It's about asking pointed questions and taking a stance indicative of a desire to invite the patient to be an active participant in their care. This doesn't have to take extra time; but it does require judicious use of the time together.

POLYPHARMACY

"Psychiatric patients are over-medicated." I hear that a lot, particularly from people who learn that I write a Psychopharmacology blog. Part of me agrees, yet another part of me realizes that this is not a simple black-or-white issue; instead, it is nuanced and complex.

There is no consistent definition of polypharmacy in the literature. So what is it, really? How many medications are too many? The most accurate definition of polypharmacy I've come across is, "the administration of many drugs together." As to how many medications are too many, there is no single number that represents the tipping point between an acceptable number of drug therapies and a "poly" issue. What's more, no medical condition presents the same way in every patient. Complications and co-morbidities are the rule, not the exception.

The core issue here is not how polypharmacy is defined or the number of medications employed. What is most important is whether the use of multiple drug treatments carries an accompanying therapeutic benefit that manifests discernable symptom improvement in the affected patient. Sometimes, it doesn't because at the first sign of treatment resistance, some prescribers find it necessary to design highly complex drug regimens without a clear rationale or good data, thereby adopting a "make it up as you go" approach. Fueled by a "more is more" belief system, these prescribers tinker with a patient's drug regimen to excess.

But polypharmacy can be beneficial by providing more therapeutic options to help patients achieve better outcomes. Too many descriptions of polypharmacy carry negative connotations, such as increased costs, poorer compliance and greater risks of side effects and drug interactions. While these negatives are indeed real, they are not the case for the majority of medicated patients. That is, most patients are medication compliant, only a relatively small number of drug-drug interactions are important, and generic alternatives for the most commonly prescribed medications are ever increasing.

Multiple medications may be necessary to effectively manage mental health disorders accompanied by physical health problems and other co-morbidities. For example, a patient with bipolar disorder, diabetes and hypertension may require as many as nine drugs to successfully manage these three disease states concurrently. Some would argue that the goal should be to decrease the number of medications this patient takes, but it could be that the person truly needs nine medications.

The most important consideration in medication management is to conceptualize a reason for each drug choice. If, after thorough analysis of a patient's drug regimen, reasons for the use of certain medications are not apparent, then the patient (or the patient's advocate) should be encouraged to ask the prescriber for a re-examination of the medication profile. Seeking a second opinion may also be warranted.

With continued advances in pharmacological therapies and an ever-increasing pool of medications from which prescribers can choose, polypharmacy will become an even more significant issue in the future. The line between just enough and too much will no doubt be further blurred.

CHAPTER 18

Psychopharmacology Going Forward

Where Psychopharmacology heads in the future will be largely dependent upon how realistically it defines its goals. Given the multidimensional nature and complexity of what influences depression, is it at all reasonable to conclude that an antidepressant, or for that matter, any other medicinal substance will be able to arrest it, or at the least, manage it better than the agents available today? What about bipolar disorder? What is it? For sure, not a single medication introduced to treat this disorder outperforms lithium day in and day out. And lithium made its debut in the late 1940s. Then there is anxiety and insomnia. It's quite evident that benzodiazepines are more than capable of reducing the excitability driven by fight-or-flight exacerbation and that there is a veritable host of sedating psychotropics capable of sledgehammering people to sleep. So people are pharmacologically calmed, is that all? As for schizophrenia and its multiple effects on different regions of the brain, can medication possibly ever effectively manage positive, negative and cognitive symptoms?

What needs to happen going forward? Here's my assessment of where Psychopharmacology is now and where this discipline needs to go.

DEPRESSION AND ANTIDEPRESSANTS

The chemical imbalance theory is on its last legs. There are entirely too many people deemed clinically depressed who don't have measurably low serotonin levels; and the plausibility of this theory is also challenged by low overall remission rates among antidepressant users. A shift to an expanded understanding of depression needs to move increasingly toward viewing it as a physical disorder. Further exploration of the depression-inflammation connection is currently the most reasonable direction to pursue. And while genotyping and phenotyping are worthy ventures in the search for reliable biomarkers in depression, such work will continue to be held hostage to the vagaries of funding. Also, the complexity of the brain often has scientists changing their minds.

193

As for antidepressants, research and development has certainly delivered on getting agents to the marketplace that are more tolerable—the major gain in this industry space. The SSRIs, SNRIs and other contemporary antidepressants are no more therapeutically effective than the pioneer Cyclic and MAOI classes, but unlike these older generation agents, there are fewer debilitating and annoying side effects.

Current antidepressants are more similar than different and truly novel, new drug chemistry has not been forthcoming, so the current group suffers from sameness. They are all slow to work, testing the patience of the already vulnerable user. And lured by hope, many folks simply take them too long, develop tolerance, underestimate the difficulties associated with withdrawal and find they are unable to get off the merry-go-round of going from one drug to another to another. Antidepressants have alleviated misery for millions of users for over 60 years, but depression is likely far too complex for a pill to solve—regardless of how novel future agents may be.

BIPOLAR DISORDER AND MOOD STABILIZERS

This particular area of psychiatric diagnosis and treatment has been stuck in neutral for some time now. The etiology of the disorder remains quite the conundrum and neuroscience has not been able to adequately address this so as to have a positive impact on future direction. There are no animal models with validity so diagnosis is all over the place, and there is no consensus on neuropathology, thus pharmacology is all over the place.

Lithium and the anticonvulsant Depakote (divalproex) work reasonably well for mania under competent care. Second-generation antipsychotics have merely been repurposed and are not considered first-line agents for mania. The real stickler when it comes to treating this disorder is its depressive phase, as traditional, contemporary antidepressants are all but failures for managing bipolar depression, so this is likely the role that antipsychotics will fill.

Pharmacological treatment creativity seems to be a must with bipolar disorder, and polypharmacy is not only necessary but warranted. Bipolar disorder is not nearly as well understood as unipolar depression, so the more light that advances in neurobiological discovery can shed into this dark space, the easier it will be for novel drug deliveries to emerge.

ANXIETY AND ANXIOLYTICS

A certain amount of anxiety is simply a part of the human condition. We all have it from time-to-time—albeit brief and merely circumstantial for some, yet chronic for others. Anxiety is hitting on all cylinders when someone hands over control to it and increasingly avoids people, places and situations that stoke it and provoke it. Outside of moments or periods of startling, imminent danger or threat, most anxiety is happening between the ears; so it is best treated by challenging the self-limiting beliefs that give birth to it.

Anxiolytics such as the benzodiazepines work for most, but at what cost? The absence of anxiety, which can manifest as euphoria with increasing doses of these medications, paves the way for misuse, abuse, tolerance, dependence and drug-seeking as a primary goal. Withdrawal can be hell. Sleep agents deliver on getting people to sleep but falter on keeping them asleep. And they are plagued by the potentially dangerous ramifications of sleepwalking as well as eating and driving without full, conscious awareness.

This space doesn't need any more players. Anxiety and insomnia have to be faced, not numbed. There will be new contenders for sure in this lucrative "discomfort" market.

Psychosis and Antipsychotics

We are many orders of magnitude away from sufficiently understanding schizophrenia and its cousins. The psychotic spectrum remains highly stigmatized; sufferers are often feared, and society struggles with making sense of its attendant array of aberrant behaviors.

Medication is effective for managing positive symptoms, but less so for negative and cognitive spectrum symptoms. And antipsychotics do virtually nothing for schizophrenia characteristics such as feelings of alienation, inadequacy and isolation. Future medication entries into this arena will have to spread their wings to provide more encompassing symptom coverage. The newer, second-generation antipsychotics, like their first-generation predecessors, can be horrible to take. Side effects are as long as an adult arm and are highlighted by medical issues such as an increased risk of type 2 diabetes, elevated cholesterol and lipids and significant weight gain, thereby bringing physical complications into play. New medications just cannot carry this kind of baggage.

ADHD and Psychostimulants

Every psychiatric syndrome on the planet adversely affects attention in some way, making it just way too easy to go to ADHD as a diagnosis without discriminating assessment. And diagnosticians are taking advantage of this in droves. Stimulants are prime candidates for diversion and find their way into the hands of people intent on abusing them for their euphoric benefits or using them as brain boosters.

Clearly and definitively, psychostimulants work and make life less hard for the accurately diagnosed. The medication field in this domain is saturated; the success of new developments would best hinge upon ease of administration—delivery systems that include more extended-release liquids for those in need of dosage fine tuning and additional patch formulations.

Regardless of future direction, psychopharmacology serves us best when it recognizes the importance of the human element in psychiatric treatment and acknowledges that many aspects of caring for those with mental illness doesn't necessarily have to include chemicals.

APPENDIX I

Making a Medication Referral

Throughout the many years I have practiced psychotherapy, the area where I still often encounter client resistance is in the use of medication to augment therapy treatment. When it comes to medication, clients will make their own choices, on their own terms, and in their own time.

Here are a few indicators to take into account when considering a referral for psychotropic medication with a patient:

- The patient is not responding favorably to psychotherapy, despite an adequate trial period. For me, this is number one.
- The patient has a complicated medical history and is taking multiple medications. Never underestimate the negative influence that certain medical disorders and some prescription medications can have on client improvement.
- The patient hasn't had a thorough physical examination in years. There may be an undiagnosed medical condition that is impinging upon what the client sought treatment for in the first place.
- The patient initially presents with prominent mood and behavior instabilities, or mood and behavior become more markedly labile as psychotherapy continues.
- The patient exhibits active and identifiable psychotic features. This is evidence of a biologically based disorder, for which pharmacological intervention is the mainstay of treatment, with psychotherapy as an adjunct to patient care.
- The patient has a personal history or significant family history of mental disturbance. Many of the disorders discussed in this book are highly heritable. Genetic predispositions are often associated with neurochemical deficits in the brain that may have an adverse influence on sustained symptom improvement unless pharmacotherapy is considered.

- There is a co-occurring substance abuse disorder. Substance abuse complicates every aspect of the medication management of mental health disorders. It can interfere with drug action, serum levels, efficacy and exacerbate the side effects of prescribed medications.

Even when one or more of the above indicators are present, mental health clinicians at all levels of experience know that getting a client on the road toward a psychotropic medication evaluation is not necessarily easy. Many clients assess the odds associated with considering alternative treatment options for some time before actually committing to the behaviors that drive the initiation of the change process. Therefore, a client's decision to follow through with a medication referral may be long and drawn out.

Often, clients are only willing to <u>consider</u> taking psychotropic medication, as opposed to actually start taking it. Client ambivalence, therefore, is a common occurrence. When facing such ambivalence, clinicians should take the opportunity to continue strengthening the therapeutic relationship. Patience is the key here. Any attempt to rush the client into a premature decision is likely to backfire and could also compromise the relationship.

Of course, waiting for clients to decide does not mean the clinician must withhold their opinion. On the contrary, if the professional knows that evidence-based literature supports a pharmacological treatment of the client's condition (for example, bipolar disorder), then they should convey that information to the client. Offering reading material or Web addresses can also help ensure that clients have as much information as possible. In this way, the client can make an informed choice regarding their future treatment. Clinicians should encourage their clients - and the clients' family members— to ask questions. Straightforward answers help to demystify the decision-making process.

Once clients have made the decision to pursue medication as a treatment option, it's important for them to understand that they have to empower themselves to benefit from physician office visits and shouldn't accept a psychiatric diagnosis from someone who barely knows them. They should ask questions, expect clear, unambiguous answers and seek other opinions if warranted. Here is a short list of important questions clients <u>should</u> be asking their prescribers:

1. What do you believe is wrong with me?
2. What might be causing this?

3. What else could it be?

4. Is there more than one treatment for what I'm experiencing?

5. Would you please tell me about the medication(s) you're prescribing?

Suggest placing these questions and others on a 3×5 index card to help with "white coat brain lock," a phenomenon characterized by forgetfulness and a lack of focus experienced by some patients when in the presence of physicians or other prescribers in a position of authority.

Frequently Asked Questions

Q. Why do so many antidepressants seem to cause sexual dysfunction?

A. In addition to its antidepressant effects, serotonin is a rather powerful vasoconstrictor. It can restrict blood flow to sexual organs and negatively impact sexual performance, libido and the ability to reach orgasm.

Q. What is the safety profile of the SSRIs?

A. From a "potential for overdose" perspective, they are actually incredibly safe. Death by SSRI overdose, according to some published reports, occurs in only about two out of every 1 million individuals using them.

Q. Is Prozac's long half-life a drawback to its action?

A. Yes and no. Prozac's long half-life can be an advantage to the individual prone to forget doses, but a disadvantage to those taking additional medications (and not only psychotropics). For example, Prozac has been reported to increase the effect of the cyclic antidepressant Norpramin (desipramine) by 400-fold in some subjects! It can also increase the effects of some benzodiazepines.

Q. How does Cymbalta differ from Effexor?

A. Both are classified as serotonin/norepinephrine reuptake inhibitors (SNRIs). However, Cymbalta is a more potent reuptake inhibitor of these neurotransmitters, and it has garnered FDA approval for the management of diabetic neuropathic pain (diabetic neuropathy).

Q. Is the diagnosis of pediatric bipolar disorder on the rise?

A. Definitely yes. According to a commentary in the December 2007 Harvard Mental Health Letter, office visits by children diagnosed with bipolar disorder multiplied 40-fold from 1994 to 2003. The number of office visits per 100,000 children rose from 25 to 1,003 in the same period.

Q. For treating depression, are the older cyclic antidepressants as effective as the newer SSRIs, SNRIs and atypicals?

A. In my estimation, yes. Most of the cyclics are dual-action—that is, they assist at increasing the availability of norepinephrine and serotonin to the "emotional brain." And they were doing so years before the advent of the more-widely prescribed SSRIs and SNRIs.

Q. Why is Topamax linked to weight loss in some subjects?

A. Topamax is an interesting drug, to say the least. Reports indicate that it was originally developed as an anti-diabetic agent, but that didn't come to pass. There is some evidence that Topamax improves insulin sensitivity, and with better management of glucose, weight loss can occur.

Q. Are recent reports regarding sleepwalking, "sleep eating" and "sleep driving" with Ambien use true?

A. Yes, but the number of <u>reported</u> cases is still small. Nevertheless, some people using Ambien report objective evidence of having engaged in these behaviors with no recollection the next day of having done so. In rare instances, Ambien may disrupt the sleep/wake cycle in some users.

Q. Are Risperdal and Invega similar?

A. Invega is actually an active metabolite of Risperdal, thus their antipsychotic actions are similar. However, Invega has an extended-release delivery system that allows for once-daily dosing, unlike Risperdal.

Q. Is Lamictal safe for use during pregnancy?

A. Unlike its predecessors Tegretol and Depakote, Lamictal does not seem to increase the risk of major birth malformations if used during pregnancy. Still, it is advisable that it not be taken during the first trimester of pregnancy.

Q. Is Wellbutrin effective in treating ADHD?

A. Yes, although primarily as an augmenting agent to the methylphenidate and dextroamphetamine type psychostimulants, which are the mainstay of treating ADHD. Wellbutrin is also effective in treating ADHD and co-morbid depression.

Q. In treating ADHD, are there any advantages to using Vyvanse over Adderall XR?

A. Both ostensibly provide 10- to 12-hour symptom coverage. But Vyvanse needs to be completely absorbed via the gastrointestinal tract before converting to its active ingredient - d-amphetamine, thus minimizing the risk that this compound can be abused through the intranasal and intravenous route, or even smoked.

Q. Is Deplin an antidepressant?

A. No, Deplin is actually a methylfolate preparation. Depressed patients consistently have lower serum folate concentrations. Deplin helps normalize amounts of the neurotransmitters norepinephrine, serotonin and dopamine, thus enabling antidepressants to be more effective.

Q. In relationship to OCD, what is "PANDAS?"

A. PANDAS is the acronym for Pediatric Autoimmune Neuropsychiatric Disorders Associated with Streptococcal infections. This is actually a subtype of pediatric OCD, triggered by strep throat, in which the body's own immune cells attack the basal ganglia within the brain rather than the strep. PANDAS OCD is usually consistent with the <u>sudden onset</u> of OCD symptoms.

Q. Why do so many psychotropic medications seem to cause weight gain?

A. Psychiatric medications which are linked to weight gain typically slow down the metabolism of carbohydrate and fat. Also, some psychotropics, such as the antipsychotics Clozaril and Zyprexa, interfere with satiety. People taking these medications often continue to eat and eat—particularly sugars— without feeling full.

Q. Will consuming alcohol prevent or diminish the potential positive effects of an antidepressant?

A. Given the complexity of individual biochemistry, the answer to this question is difficult to nail down; but it certainly depends on the quantity and frequency of alcohol use. There are a few studies indicating that any amount of alcohol— even just one alcoholic beverage—can lead to a diminished antidepressant response. I routinely recommend to those using antidepressants that they consume no more than two (2) alcoholic beverages a week.

Q. What's the chance that there will be some untoward and unintended consequences between alcohol and antidepressants?

A. This largely depends on the actions of the antidepressant prescribed, particularly its capacity for producing sedation. There is much less concern about additive sedation if alcohol is ingested in combination with a non-sedating antidepressant. On the other hand, combining alcohol with a sedating antidepressant may lead the individual to become more intoxicated than would otherwise be anticipated.

Q. When diagnosing depression in a client, how concerned should I be about identifying specific depression subtypes?

A. The important issue here is whether labeling a depression by subtype assists the clinician in treating the client more effectively. With few exceptions, the answer is NO. Subtypes are generally poor predictors of treatment response. There are some exceptions however. Seasonal Affective Disorder may respond to light therapy as well as antidepressants, and psychotic depressions all but always require antidepressant treatment augmented with antipsychotics.

Q. How long does it take for Zoloft, Paxil, Effexor and Wellbutrin to take effect?

A. At least 50 percent of those who will eventually respond to the above mentioned antidepressants will begin to demonstrate improvement within one or two weeks of treatment initiation. Users most often report an increase in energy and productivity coupled with a decrease in sensitivity (particularly to inappropriate comments from others) and anger. Remission of mood symptoms is tougher. Because depression is neurotoxic, this may span over an 8–12 week period.

Q. Should adults take ADHD drugs?

A. Absolutely adults should take them. Seventy percent of those diagnosed with ADD in childhood or adolescence go on to experience symptoms in adulthood. If untreated, these adults will struggle with distractibility and inattention throughout their entire lives.

Q. Is bipolar disorder more difficult to diagnose in children than in adults?

A. Yes, bipolar disorder is actually very hard to diagnose in children mostly because of the high incidence of multiple co-existing disorders with symptom overlap seen in children. The prime example of a co-existing condition with symptom overlap is ADHD. Two of the symptoms presumed to be evidence of a mood disorder (bipolar)—irritability and hyperactivity—are also key criteria for an ADHD diagnosis. Another issue complicating the diagnosis of bipolar disorder in children is that there is no consensus on how to measure symptom severity. If a child is perceived as disruptive, it could be that his or her behavior deviates wildly from the mean, or it could be that the diagnosing clinician(s) is overly intolerant of unruly behavior.

Q. What are the biggest risk factors for developing depression?

A. The three biggest risk factors are: (1) Genetic predisposition. Many that meet criteria for major depressive disorder have a significant family history for depression. (2) Environmental events. Those that have recently experienced situational factors such as the death of a loved one, a recent divorce or a job loss are at risk for developing depression. (3) Physical illness. Physical illnesses such as diabetes and hypothyroidism are major contributors to depressive symptom emergence.

Q. Are women more likely to develop depression than men? Why or why not?

A. Women are twice as likely to develop depression compared to men. It is a myth that this is primarily a hormonal issue or that women produce less serotonin than men. Instead women are at twice the risk due to discrimination, poverty, oppression and the stresses of single parenthood.

Q. Are there certain ethnicities that are more likely to be depressed than others?

A. Approximately 30 percent of Hispanics report suffering depression compared to 26 percent for whites, 20 percent for blacks, and 16 percent for Asians. However, approximately 75 percent of whites with self-reported depression go on to receive an official diagnosis vs. 62 percent for Hispanics, 58 percent for blacks and 47 percent for Asians.

Q. Is ADHD being over diagnosed or underdiagnosed?

A. The answer is both. Over diagnosis is an issue because academic expectations of American children are rising and occurring at an earlier age. Children are expected to sit longer, concentrate more, stay focused and read and write earlier. Also, class sizes are increasing at the same time teachers are expected to meet the needs of every child. Parents are also stressed. Children are hurried from one activity to another. There is less family time. All of these factors contribute to a child not focusing and paying attention. But ADHD is also underdiagnosed. A child can be labeled as "bad" when he continually engages in a behavior that is viewed as purposeful and within his control. This child is then often asked to "try harder," which is actually outside of his control.

Q. Is depression contagious?

A. In the sense that depression can be "caught" like the flu bug— the answer is no. But if you are continuously around sad, angry or fearful people you may find yourself starting to feel that way. That's because we are all vulnerable to absorbing negativity. But there's a big difference between absorbing depression-like symptoms and being actually clinically depressed. Anyone who is regularly in the company of a clinically depressed person should empower themselves to understand depression as an illness and should also strive to get their own needs met.

Q. What questions should clients ask when having a psychiatric medication evaluation?

A. Many clients develop "white-coat brain lock" when it comes to asking questions—particularly on the first visit—because one of the most prevalent communication gaps is between doctors and patients. On a 3×5 index card, have your client write down the following five questions and recommend that they ask these after the doctor has completed the initial assessment and has evaluated the client's history and presenting symptoms:

1. "What do you think is wrong with me?"
2. "What might be causing this?"
3. "What else could it be?"
4. "Is there more than one treatment for my disorder?"
5. "Would you please tell me about the medication(s) you're prescribing for me?"

The average length of a general practice physician office visit nowadays is seven (7) minutes; so as simple as they may be, these questions often go unanswered due to the flurry of activity in physicians' offices. So clients have to empower themselves to maximize the benefits of office visits. And an empowered client is usually a <u>compliant</u> client.

Q. Can patients with a long history of panic attacks and depression as well benefit from antidepressants?

A. Sure. The SSRI antidepressants have anti-anxiety benefits as well as antidepressant effects. Because of their slow onset of action, they are less effective for the acute onset symptoms of panic and more effective for the maintenance treatment of panic symptoms.

APPENDIX III

Medication Noncompliance and How Healthcare Professionals Can Help

The basic definition of noncompliance is the failure to take medication according to prescribed directions. But it's more than non-adherence to directions, noncompliance is also indicative of the misuse of medication. Here are five common causes of noncompliance and how healthcare professionals can help.

- **Side Effects**. In a "perfect drug" scenario, medications would zero in on their intended target systems generating only desired, therapeutic effects, then metabolize and leave the body. Unfortunately, it's not that simple, as medications produce unintended consequences as well.

- **How healthcare professionals can help:** It is important to be honest with clients about side effects. Point out that although practically every drug—prescription and over-the-counter—has side effects, many of them are short-lived and "run their course," so to speak, after the body adapts to the new substance. Discuss the typical side effects of the medications that the client is taking, and suggest ways for combating them. For example, drugs that are associated with the side effects of anxiety and insomnia are best taken in the morning. Sedating medications should be taken at bedtime and those linked to nausea are to be consumed on a full stomach.

- **Cost.** Unfortunately, most brand name medications are outrageously expensive nowadays. So it is no surprise that the poor and particularly the elderly on fixed incomes are prone to breaking their medications in half or taking them every other day. As important as medication may be to quality of life and even survival, it's not high in the pecking order when it comes to one's hierarchy of needs.

- **How healthcare professionals can help:** The place to start is with the client's choice of insurance company or plan. Help them find out about the range of prescription benefits and whether or not the medications they are taking are covered under their plan. Clarify co-pay information and whether or not brand name drugs are covered. This is particularly important if they're taking several medications. Suggest comparison-shopping among several pharmacies. There are often significant price differences for the same drug from pharmacy to pharmacy. Check out the website *www.drugcoupons.com* for coupons that can be used for medications. A number of assistance programs are available through states, nonprofits and drug companies. Contact the Partnership for Prescription Assistance *www.pparx.org* for eligibility requirements. PPA helps the uninsured or those struggling financially to gain access to assistance programs that are either free or very low cost. Find out if the client's physician is willing to prescribe either a less expensive brand of the medication they are taking or a generic. More and more pharmacies have followed Wal-Mart's lead and are offering some generics for as little as $4.00 per prescription. The purchase of prescriptions via mail order, particularly in larger quantities, offers handsome savings in many instances.

- **Forgetfulness.** Forgetting to take medication according to prescribed directions is the most common cause of noncompliance. It is often the result of poor organization, memory compromise and sometimes downright obstinace, that is, some people "conveniently" forget.

- **How healthcare professionals can help:** Compartmentalized pillboxes, medication calendars, post-it note reminders, timers and even high tech talking devices that sound an alarm when a dose is missed are all helpful. Help clients set up a strategy for taking medications at the same time every day and enlist the help of family members whenever possible. Available and supportive family members can either administer medication directly to the client or remind them via a phone call. The key here is to set up a clockwork pattern of daily repetition for the consumption of medication.

- **"The I'm Cured Syndrome."** Way too many people treat prescribed medication as they would a Tylenol for a simple, uncomplicated tension headache. That is, once they either begin to feel better or their symptoms remit, they abruptly stop or gradually discontinue the drug. The reasoning for this action, albeit illogical, is simple. Most people want to be done with medication as quickly as possible because it is viewed as a necessary evil. For many, having to take medication serves as an ever-present reminder of something undesirable, such as a physical illness or mental disorder.

- **How healthcare professionals can help:** This one can be tough and is at times met with resistance. But clients need to be reminded that medication is a vehicle that has fostered improvement in the first place, and that abrupt or gradual discontinuation isn't warranted without the approval or recommendation from the client's prescriber. Some clients need to bluntly hear that this is a matter they shouldn't take into their own hands.

- **Frequency of Use.** This is a rather linear issue. The more times per day someone has to take a medication, the greater the frequency of a missed dose. It's that simple. There's also a" multiplier effect" associated with frequency of use that is exacerbated in the client taking multiple medications. This can make for a real mess.

- **How healthcare professionals can help:** Research whether the client's medication is possibly available in a once-daily formulation. If so, guide them via recommendations as to how they can advocate with the prescriber on their own behalf for once-daily preparations; or with a properly executed release, contact the prescriber directly for them. It can be particularly important for the professional to initiate contact with the prescriber on behalf of elderly clients or for those who are reticent about doing so themselves. If not available, the aforementioned clockwork pattern of medication use that fosters a cycle of daily repetition becomes even more important.

APPENDIX IV

Are All Drugs Created Equal?
Brand Name vs. Generic Medications

Are low-priced generic medications as safe and effective as their brand name counterparts? It depends on whom you're asking, comparative studies, biases and personal experience. All four of these issues figure prominently into determining the answer to this question. Here's more detail:

- **Whom you ask:** Ask a brand name drug manufacturer, and they will obviously claim that their medications are better than generics. After all, brand name drugs are subject to rigorous FDA clinical trials and are tested more thoroughly on patients than generics. When FDA approved, brand name drugs reap price benefits and patent protection for as long as 20 years. Prices for brand name drugs reflect the steep research and development expenditures associated with developing, testing and getting drugs to market, the companies say. But ask a manufacturer of generic medicines, and they will say their products are every bit as effective as their brand name counterparts. This is because the FDA <u>requires</u> generics to be "bioequivalent." This means the generic medication must contain the same active ingredients as the brand name equivalent, and when taken by patients, they must also produce similar results. Therefore, one should expect a generic to be as safe and effective as a brand name medication.

- **Comparative studies:** In a recent study published in the *Journal of the American Medical Association*, researchers compared generic and brand name drugs for the treatment of heart and artery disease. They studied beta blockers, diuretics, statins (for high LDL cholesterol) and warfarin (a blood thinner)—some of the most commonly prescribed medications worldwide. Thirty eight of the studies were randomized controlled trials—indicative of high reliability. Of these 38 studies, 36 found no

213

real difference between generic and brand. Yet some physicians remain concerned. They point out that the bioequivalence studies used by the FDA to make its determinations aren't made public. As a result, doctors have no way of knowing when the FDA has found a difference; nor do they know how telling that difference, if any, might be. Physicians are also unable to learn about differences in fillers and other additives, which might change the rates of release. Perhaps that's why only 12 of 43 medical journal commentaries on the subject encourage the use of generics.

- **Biases:** Biases tend to be influenced by our belief systems, and they exist in practically every area of our lives. Medication is no exception. If you are the CEO of a pharmaceutical company, you're likely biased in favor of brand name drugs. If on the other hand, you are living on a fixed income and have encountered no ill effects from generics, it is likely you will favor them.

- **Personal experience:** Previous experience weighs heavily on future choices and decisions. For example, if a patient switches from a brand name drug to a generic drug and notices no difference in their health, they will likely believe that generics can be readily substituted for brand name products. But if the same patient experienced new side effects or diminished effectiveness with the generic medication, they might be more skeptical of the switch. In both cases, the person's opinion would have been affected by their personal experience. Further, this is essentially anecdotal evidence based on a sample of just one person, and therefore unscientific. Similarly, the way physicians view generic medications often is closely associated with the experiences of their patients. In today's medical environment, prescribing habits have changed. Most physicians either accept or have been influenced into generic substitution by the rigorous, cost-conscious practices of third-party insurers. If a patient complains though, doctors will usually not hesitate to change a prescription back to its brand name version.

- **The bottom line:** Placing personal accounts, comparative studies, biases and experiences aside, the FDA is satisfied with the performance of generic drugs.

The Placebo Effect

The placebo effect is likely as old as the healing professions themselves. In the classic placebo effect, a person <u>consciously</u> believes that a substance is therapeutic, and this belief generates a positive effect on medical or psychological symptom improvement. Over the centuries, doctors have purposely used inactive substances when they had no suitable medications to treat certain medical maladies. In numerous field trials, people in placebo groups have been found to improve at least as much as people in drug groups through the conscious belief that what they received generated a positive effect on their medical or psychological symptom improvement. Specifically, placebos have demonstrated positive results in the treatment of depression, pain, asthma, arthritis, hypertension, insomnia and other conditions. Placebos have even been found to produce a positive response when the person knows they are taking a placebo.

For several decades however, scientists and researchers have known that placebo effects can also arise from <u>subconscious</u> associations. Any stimuli that a patient may link with symptom improvement—a physician's white lab coat a physical examination, the touch of the stethoscope to the chest, even the smell of alcohol in the examining room—may induce positive physiological responses. This can be true even when a patient has no explicit belief or faith in the treatment being administered.

The placebo effect probably accounts for most of the benefits associated with treatments such as acupuncture, aromatherapy, homeopathy and other alternative treatments. It also accounts for success with more conventional treatments. For example half of all responses to antidepressants are attributable to the placebo effect, according to the American Psychological Association. Other estimates place the placebo response rate for antidepressants as high as 73 percent.

Conditions linked to significant psychological distress are <u>most</u> likely to respond to placebo. Some possible mechanisms for this are as follows:

- Psychological theory—psychology affects biology, beliefs affect biochemistry, the old "if you want to change the way you feel, change the way you think" adage.
- Nature takes its course—we often get better by doing nothing at all, allowing the body to heal itself.
- Process of treatment—touching (when appropriate), displaying a caring attitude, being attentive and communicating effectively—may elicit a placebo response.

  Using the placebo effect:

- Inspire patient confidence by acting and dressing professionally.
- Display symbols of comfort in your office. These may include soothing artwork, positive affirmations, or the gentle sound of water trickling from a "mini-fountain."
- Discreetly take notes during meetings. This of course indicates attentiveness and that the clinician is immersed in the patient's condition. Patients equate note taking with a clinician who will study their case, and this intensifies their belief that a positive outcome is likely.
- Lean slightly forward when addressing the patient and asking questions. Leaning forward is a gesture of interest in the patient's problem. Patients equate this with a clinician who is empathic and cares about them.
- Solicit patient beliefs and input when selecting treatment interventions.
- Most important, instill <u>hope</u> and <u>optimism</u> when discussing the prognosis of the presenting problem.

Finally, consider that the color of a tablet can add a placebo boost to the physiological effects in real, legitimate drugs. For example, yellow pills tend to make the most effective antidepressants—like doses of drug-induced sunshine. Green tablets or capsules reduce anxiety—looking out over a plush landscape is soothing and the dominant green color scheme is obvious to us all. And red tablets are associated with a stimulating kick and "charged-up" sensation.

The placebo response couldn't care less if the impetus for healing is due to pharmacological success, a caring clinician or an injection of saline. All it requires is someone with a reasonable expectation of getting better. That is powerful medicine!

Tapering and Discontinuing Psychotropic Medication

More and more calls and e-mails are filtering into my office these days from people interested in tapering and discontinuing psychotropic medication. My first two questions to them are why and, why now? Answers to these questions typically align with three themes: 1) The users believe the drug(s) isn't helping them anymore, 2) They'd like to try going it alone without medication, and 3) They don't want to run the risk of long-term dependence on medication, particularly with benzodiazepines and sleeping pills.

All three of these responses are reasonable and valid, so then I follow up with these questions: How equipped are you for doing this, specifically, have you thought about or do you have a plan for managing the tough moments that will inevitably occur once you get started? How susceptible are you to relapse? Can you see this all the way through without looking back? These questions render some people speechless or deliver answers that indicate potential pitfalls haven't been adequately considered.

Then there's the even bigger picture as to which psychotropic medication classes can be successfully tapered or discontinued. Credible literature is sparse when it comes to tapering mood stabilizers for bipolar disorder and antipsychotics for the psychotic spectrum. And there is virtually no mention of discontinuing these medications for long periods, as these disorders are associated with lifetime prevalence. Even the psychostimulants for ADHD are used for long stretches of time—subject to tapering only, without discontinuation. This leaves the antidepressants and the anxiolytics—particularly the benzodiazepines and sleep agents.

The literature supports a trial off antidepressant medications after a year of full recovery from moderate depression and consideration of long-term use after a second relapse. What about after years of antidepressant use, though? This question hasn't been studied in any measurable detail, thus tapering and discontinuation remain quite the conundrum for the individual using antidepressants for a decade or longer.

As for the benzodiazepines, operatively these drugs should be used for no longer than a few weeks, and in rare instances for up to six months, although these time frames are routinely violated.

TAPERING AND DISCONTINUATION OF ANTIDEPRESSANTS, BENZODIAZEPINES, AND SLEEP AGENTS

There's no ONE right way of tapering and discontinuing these drug classes, no algorithm or formula guaranteeing success, and there are countless opinions and recommendations on how to proceed. The key variables associated with getting started are how long the drug has been used, at what dose, and its pharmacokinetics—particularly the drug's half-life. These factors will influence the intensity of the withdrawal symptoms most commonly associated with these medication classes—flu-like symptoms, electric shock sensations in the hands and feet, brain zapping and possible seizures.

Antidepressants, and most certainly the benzodiazepines, as well as the sleep drugs Ambien, Lunesta etc. should <u>never be stopped abruptly.</u> At sub-therapeutic or suboptimal dosing, practically anyone should be able to safely proceed toward discontinuation within two months. At customary, maximum or excessively high daily dosage ranges, the tapering process should proceed in a manner that best suits the individual's tolerance for discomfort. The single most important factor is for the patient to proceed at a slow but steady pace to avoid becoming discouraged and subsequently aborting the entire process.

Here's an example describing a slow, safe and effective way of tapering the benzodiazepine Valium (diazepam), used in this instance, for insomnia:

A 42-year-old female has been taking Valium (diazepam) 20mg per night for insomnia for approximately two years. The recommendation for tapering this dose with discontinuation as the eventual goal is as follows: She is to begin the taper by reducing the 20mg per night dose by 2.5mg on one (1) night per week. It is suggested that she begin on a night prior to a day when she has less responsibilities. She begins on a Friday night by taking 17.5 mg of Valium (diazepam). Then the following week she is to reduce the 20mg nightly dose by 2.5mg on another night of the week—avoiding two nights in a row at first. She is to then continue reducing by 2.5mg until she's taking 17.5mg per night, every night of the week. She is instructed to continue with this tapering cycle—reducing by 2.5mg until taking 15mg per night, then 12.5mg per night and so on. Successful completion, defined as 0mg nightly, will take a bit over one year if the plan is followed and adhered to correctly.

Finally, no one should begin doing this without consulting their physician or prescriber. The prescriber should decide on and initiate the tapering and discontinuation plan and be kept informed every step of the way, particularly if things become problematic. And the patient should keep an eye on the prize—saying goodbye to drugs that once served a purpose but have now outlived their usefulness.

Pharmacogenetic Testing in Psychiatry

The evaluation and assessment process in psychiatry typically goes something like this: A patient enters the treating clinician's office and is asked a series of questions pursuant to their presenting problem. Based on the answers provided, additional questions – in the form of a questionnaire or the use of a clinical scale – may be utilized to ascertain additional information. Then there's usually a discussion with the patient regarding the findings, a diagnosis (or at least a preliminary one) is put forth, and in collaboration with the patient, a treatment plan is suggested. Pretty straightforward, right? Well, the mystery often begins when medication use enters the picture as part of the treatment going forward.

Drug prescribing has long been a trial-and-error phenomenon in both physical and psychiatric medicine. Physical medicine though has this advantage: science has provided us a whole lot more information about the body than it has about the brain, and this bears itself out in the track record of certain psychiatric medication classes. With antidepressants for example, only 30 percent of users will experience some measurable symptom relief after their first antidepressant trial. This is because trial-and-error prescribing doesn't account for the genetic variabilities and biochemical makeup differences among us, so what works for one depressed patient may very well not work for another. Therefore, knowledge of a patient's genetic background can aid clinicians in providing a more "personalized" medication strategy by predicting both drug response and tolerability. Clinicians can then use this information to make up for a gene defect or to adjust drug dosage to assist the rate at which a patient metabolizes different medications. This intervention is called *Pharmacogenetic testing* and it's upon us.

There are several commercial outlets that sell pharmacogenetic tests for psychiatric applications. They include Genomind, Pathway Genomics, Genelex, Assurex Health, Genecept and GeneSight Psychotropic. The prices for these gene panels range from $99 on the low end to hundreds of dollars at the top end, and there is no strong push to influence insurance companies to pony up for these tests at this time.

The sixty-four-dollar question though is: does this information lead to better clinical outcomes? A couple of studies have reported that GeneSight Psychotropic was effective for managing patients with depression – although there were methodological issues with patient assignment to study groups. In addition, prescribers and patients were not fully blinded, potentially influencing a placebo effect to occur, which could reflect improved outcomes for those getting the testing. Also, genetic makeup is but a small part of drug response and tolerability, with other issues serving as strong contributors. Substances such as tobacco and dietary supplements may interfere with the metabolism of antidepressants for example, and metabolic issues involving age, the disease process and gender can also affect how someone responds to certain drugs. Therefore, genetic and nongenetic determinants apply.

As of this writing, pharmacogenetics is not ready for prime time, it's expensive and this testing industry is significantly underregulated, in that companies don't have to prove the validity of their tests before marketing and selling them. It is however, an exciting and intriguing development for psychiatry.

The art of clinical practice as it relates to prescribing medication will always hinge on establishing a clear rationale for drug use in the first place, but pharmacogenetic testing can likely help by shedding light on risk factors affecting some patients because of their individual biochemistry. These patients may benefit from closer and more frequent follow-up.

If risk can be classified and if these tests, through further refinement, are able to provide some sense of how patients are likely to do on medication treatment, this would be quite an advance.

Master Drug Chart

Brand Name	Generic Name
Abilify	aripiprazole
Adapin	doxepin
Adderall	dextroamphetamine/amphetamine
Adderall XR	dextroamphetamine/amphetamine
Ambien	zolpidem
Anafranil	clomipramine
Aplenzin	bupropion Hbr
Asendin	amoxapine
Atarax	hydroxyzine
Ativan	lorazepam
Aventyl	nortriptyline
Belsomra	suvorexant
Brintellix	vortioxetine
BuSpar	buspirone
Catapres	clonidine
Celexa	citalopram
Centrax	prazepam
Clozaril	clozapine
Concerta	methylphenidate
Cymbalta	duloxetine
Daytrana	methylphenidate
Depakote	divalproex
Desyrel	trazodone
Dexedrine	dextroamphetamine
Dexedrine	dextroamphetamine

Brand Name	Generic Name
Dextrostat	dextroamphetamine
Edular	zolpidem tartrate
Effexor	venlafaxine
Effexor SR	venlafaxine SR
Elavil	amitriptyline
Emsam (transdermal)	selegiline
Eskalith	lithium carbonate
Fanapt	iloperidone
Fetzima	levomilnacipran
Focalin	dexmethylphenidate
Focalin XR	dexmethylphenidate XR
Gabitril	tiagabine
Geodon	ziprasidone
Haldol	haloperidol
Inderal	propranolol
Intermezzo	zolpidem sublingual
Intuniv	guanfacine LA
Invega	paliperidone
Klonopin	clonazepam
Lamictal	lamotrigine
Latuda	lurasidone
Lexapro	escitalopram
Librium	chlordiazepoxide
Loxitane	loxapine
Ludiomil	maprotiline
Lunesta	eszopiclone
Luvox	fluvoxamine
Mellaril	thioridazine
Metadate CD	methylphenidate
Methylin	methylphenidate
Moban	molindone
Nardil	phenelzine
Navane	thiothixene
Neurontin	gabapentin

Brand Name	Generic Name
Norpramin	desipramine
Oleptro	trazodone extended-release
Orap	pimozide
Pamelor	nortriptyline
Parnate	tranylcypromine
Paxil	paroxetine
Pristiq	desvenlafaxine
Prolixin	fluphenazine
Prozac	fluoxetine
Quillivant XR	methylphenidate oral suspension
Remeron	mirtazapine
Risperdal	risperidone
Ritalin	methylphenidate
Ritalin LA	methylphenidate LA
Ritalin SR	methylphenidate SR
Rozerem	ramelteon
Saphris	asenapine
Sarafem	fluoxetine
Serax	oxazepam
Serentil	mesoridazine
Seroquel	quetiapine
Sinequan	doxepin
Sonata	zaleplon
Stelazine	trifluoperazine
Strattera	atomoxetine
Surmontil	trimipramine
Symbyax	olanzapine/fluoxetine
Tegretol	carbamazepine
Tenex	guanfacine
Tenormin	atenolol
Thorazine	chlorpromazine
Tofranil	imipramine
Topamax	topiramate
Tranxene	clorazepate

Brand Name	**Generic Name**
Trilafon	perphenazine
Trileptal	oxcarbazepine
Valium	diazepam
Viibryd	vilazodone
Vistaril	hydroxyzine
Vivactil	protriptyline
Vyvanse	lisdexamfetamine
Wellbutrin	bupropion
Wellbutrin SR	bupropion LA
Wellbutrin XL	bupropion SR
Xanax	alprazolam
Zoloft	sertraline
Zyprexa	olanzapine

Resources

Agency for Healthcare Research and Quality. 2002. S-adenosyl-L- methionine for treatment of depression, osteoarthritis, and liver disease. Summary Report, AHRQ Publication No. 02-E033. Rockville, MD: Agency for Healthcare Research and Quality, ahrq.gov.

Ainsworth, P. 2000. *Understanding Depression*. Jackson, MS: University Press of Mississippi.

Akiskal, H. S. 1996. The prevalent clinical spectrum of bipolar disorders: beyond DSM-IV. *Journal of Clinical Psychopharmacology*. 16: (suppl) 4s- 14s.

American Academy of Neurology. 2008. Does Gingko Biloba Affect Memory? sciencedaily.com.

American Psychiatric Association. 1994. Diagnostic and statistical manual of mental disorders (4th ed.). Washington, DC: Author

American Psychiatric Association. 2013. Diagnostic and statistical manual of mental disorders. (5th ed.). Washington, DC: Author.

Anderson, P. 2008. Low Testosterone Levels Linked with Higher Risk of Depression. *Medscape Medical News*. medscape.com.

Antidepressants for the heart. (2002). *Harvard Mental Health Letter* 18:9.

Appleton, W. 2000. *Prozac and the New Antidepressants*. New York: Penguin Putnam, Inc.

Arato, M., C.M. Banki, G. Bissette, C.B. Nemeroff. 1989. Elevated CSF CRF in suicide victims. *Biological Psychiatry* 25(3):355–359.

Arnstein, Amy F.T. 2007. Alpha-2 agonists in the treatment of ADHD. Medscape Psychiatry & Mental Health, medscape.com.

Ashih, H. 2009. Saphris and Fanapt: Two New Antipsychotics. The Carlat Report Psychiatry. 7(12):1–2.

Beaubrun, G., and G. E. Gary. 2000. A review of herbal medicines for psychiatric disorders. *Psychiatric Services* 51(9):1130–1134.

Bender, K. J., ed. 1993. Narcotic agents for alcoholism. *Psychotropics*. 13:6–8.

Benet, L. Z., J. R. Mitchell, and L. B. Sherner. 1990a. General Principles. In *Goodman & Gilman's: The Pharmacological Basis of Therapeutics*. A. G. Gilman, T. W. Rall, A. S. Nies, and P. Taylor, eds. New York: Pergamon Press.

Bentley, K., and Walsh, J. 2001. *The Social Worker and Pyschotropic Medication*. 2nd Edition. New York: The Free Press.

Brown, S. A. and M. A. Schuckit. 1988. Changes in depression among abstinent alcoholics. *Journal of the Study of Alcoholism.* 49:412–417.

Charney, D.S., Nemeroff, C.B., Braun, S. 2004. *The Peace of Mind Prescription: An Authoritative Guide to Finding the Most Effective Treatment for Anxiety and Depression.* Boston: Houghton Mifflin.

Cowley, G., et al. 1990. A breakthrough drug for depression. *Newsweek*, March 26.

Davis, J. M. et al. A meta-analysis of the efficacy of second generation antipsychotics. *Archives of General Psychiatry 2003.* June; 60:553–64.

Diamond, R. 2002. *Instant Psychopharmacology.* 2nd Edition. New York: W. W. Norton and Company.

Does gingko biloba affect memory? (2008). Science Daily.com

Dubovsky, S. (2003). Fluoxetine safety during pregnancy and lactation. *Journal Watch Psychiatry, 9:7.*

Einarson, A. 2005. The safety of psychotropic drug use during pregnancy: a review. Medscape General Medicine. 7(4), medscape.com.

Empfield, M., Bakalar, N. 2001. *Understanding Teenage Depression: A Guide to Diagnosis, Treatment, and Management.* New York: H. Holt.

Fowler, M. 2001. *Maybe You Know My Teen: A Parent's Guide to Helping Your Adolescent with Attention Deficit Hyperactivity Disorder.* New York: Broadway Books.

Garland, T. 2014. Self-Regulation Interventions and Strategies. Eau Claire, WI: PESI Publishing & Media.

Geller, B. 2003. Serotonergic symptoms in SSRI exposed infants. *Journal Watch Psychiatry.* 9:10.

Geller, B. Antidepressants during pregnancy: benefits for children. *Journal Watch Psychiatry.* 9:1.

Ghaemi, S. N. 2000. New treatments for bipolar disorder: the role of atypical neuroleptic agents. *Journal of Clinical Psychopharmacology.* 61: (suppl)33–42.

Gitlin, M. 1996. Neurology/Psychiatry Update. *Pharmacist's Letter.* 18:3.

Gitlin, M.J. 1996. *The Psychotherapist's Guide to Psychopharmacology.* 2nd Edition. New York: Free Press.

Glazener, F. S. 1992. Adverse drug reactions. In *Melmon and Morrelli's Clinical Pharmacology: Basic Principles in Theraputics.* 3rd Edition. D. W. Nierenberg, ed. New York: McGraw-Hill.

Harvard Medical School. 2008. A SAD Story: Seasonal Affective Disorder. *Harvard Health Letter.*

Harvard University. 2003. Study Suggests Depressed Men May Benefit from Testosterone Replacement Therapy. hms.Harvard.edu/news/

Helgoe, L.A., Wilhelm, L.R., Kommor, M.J. 2005. *The Anxiety Answer Book.* Naperville, IL: Sourcebooks.

Hoffman, R.E., et al. 2000. Transcranial magnetic stimulation and auditory hallucinations in schizophrenia. *Lancet.* 355:1073–1075.

Holick, M. 2007. Vitamin D Deficiency. *N Engl J Med* 357:266–281. Jacobs, G. 1998. Say Good Night To Insomnia. New York, N.Y.: St. Martin's Press.

Jellin, J. 2002. Neurology/Psychiatry Update. *Pharmacists Letter.* 18:10.

Jellin, J. 2002. Pediatrics Update. *Pharmacists Letter.* 18:8.

Jellin, J. 2002. Psychotropic Medication Update. *The Brown University Child and Adolescent Psychopharmacology Update.* 4:10, 5:2.

Johnson, B. A. et al. 2003. Oral topiramate for treatment of alcohol dependence. *Lancet.* May 17; 261:1677–85

Kraepelin, E. 1921. *Textbook of Psychiatry,* 7th Edition. (abstracted). Translated by Diefendorf. London: MacMillan 1907.

Kramer, P.D. 1997. *Listening to Prozac: The Landmark Book About Antidepressant and the Remaking of the Self.* Revised Edition. New York: Penguin.

LaPlante, B.J. 2007. Atypical antipsychotics and bipolar disorder. Medscape Psychiatry & Mental Health, medscape.com.

Levine, D. 2014. New therapies offer bright hope against the darkness of depression. *health@ latimes.com.*

Magid, M., et al. 2014. Treatment of Major Depressive Disorder Using Botulinum Toxin A: A 24-week Randomized, Double-Blind, Placebo-Controlled Study. *Journal of Clinical Psychiatry.*75(8): 837–844

Manos, M. J. 2005. Opinions on drug holidays in pediatric ADHD. Medscape Psychiatry & Mental Health. 10(2), medscape.com.

Martin, A., Scahill, L., Charney, D., and Leckman, J. 2003. *Pediatric Psychopharmacology, Principles and Practice.* New York, NY: Oxford University Press, Inc.

Mayo Foundation for Medical Education and Research. 2006. Electroconvulsive Therapy (ECT): Treating Severe Depression and Mental Illness, mayoclinic.com.

Mays, D. 2011. Psychiatric Medications: Prescription and "Alternative." 11th Edition.

Miller, R., Mason, S.E., eds. 2002. *Diagnosis: Schizophrenia: A Comprehensive Resource for Patients, Families, and Helping Professionals.* New York: Columbia University Press.

Mintz, D. 2014. Psychodynamic Psychopharmacology. *The Carlat Report Psychiatry.* 12 (4): 8

Mischoulon, D., et al. 1999. Strategies for augmentation of SSRI treatment: a survey of an academic psychopharmacology practice. *Harvard Review of Psychiatry.* 6:322–326.

National Institute of Mental Health, National Institutes of Health. 2007. Meeting Summary: Childhood and Adolescent Onset Schizophrenia: Research Challenges and Opportunities, nimh.nih.gov.

Neziroglu, F., Yaryura-Tobias, J.A. 1997. *Over and Over Again: Understanding Obsessive-Compulsive Disorder.* San Francisco: Jossey-Bass.

Nidhino, S. E., E. Mignot, and W. C. Dement. 1998. Sedative-hypnotics. In Textbook of Psychopharmacology. 2nd Edition. A. F. Schatzberg and C. B. Nemeroff, eds. 487–502.

Osborn, I. 1998. *Tormenting Thoughts and Secret Rituals: The Hidden Epidemic of Obsessive-Compulsive Disorder.* New York: Pantheon Books.

Page, D. 2006. UCLA Develops Unique Nerve-stimulation Epilepsy Treatment, http://newsroom.ucla.edu.

Parikh, A. 2012. Diagnosis and Treatment of ADHD in Adults. Carlat Report Psychiatry. 10(2):3–5

Papolos, D., Papolos, J. 1999. *The Bipolar Child.* New York: Broadway Books.

PDR staff/editors. 2008. *Physicians' Desk Reference.* New York: Thomson Healthcare.

Peet, M., D.F. Horribin. 2002 A dose-ranging study of the effects of ethyl- eicosapentaenoate in patients with ongoing depression despite apparently adequate treatment with standard drugs. *Archives of General Psychiatry,* 59:913–919.

Perry, P. el al. 2002.Testosterone therapy in late-life major depression in males. *Journal of Clinical Psychiatry.* Dec. 63:12 1096–1101.

Pollock, V. E. 1992. Meta-analysis of subjective sensitivity to alcohol in sons of alcoholics. *American Journal of Psychiatry.*149:1534–1538.

Porter, R. 2002. *Madness: A Brief History.* Oxford, NY: Oxford University Press.

Preston, J., O'Neal, M., and Talaga, M. 2010. *Handbook of Clinical Psychopharmacology for Therapists.* 6th Edition. Oakland, CA: New Harbinger.

Puzantian, T. 2014. Belsomra: A New Hypnotic? Don't Get Too Excited. The Carlat Report Psychiatry. 12(10):5,7.

Puzantian, T. 2010. Psychotropics in Pregnancy and Breastfeeding. The Carlat Report Psychiatry. 8(11):3–4.

Rosen, L.E., Amador, X.F. 1996. *When Someone You Love is Depressed: How to Help Your Loved One without Losing Yourself.* New York: Free Press.

Roy-Byrne, P. 2003. Antidepressant effects of SAMe, Redux. Journal Watch Psychiatry. 9:1.

Roy-Byrne, P. 2003. The new ADHD drug atomoxetine: its mechanism for action. *Journal Watch Psychiatry.* 9:1.

Scherk, H., F.G. Pajonk, S. Leucht. 2007. Second-generation antipsychotic agents in the treatment of acute mania: a systematic review and meta- analysis of randomized controlled trials. *Archives of General Psychiatry.* 64(4):442–455.

Schildkraut, J. J. 1970. *Neuropsychopharmacology and the Affective Disorders* (New England Journal of Medicine Medical Progress Series). New York: Little, Brown.

Schwarz, A. 2013. ADHD. Seen in 11% of U.S. Children as Diagnoses Rise. *The New York Times Health.* nytimes.com

Stahl, S. 1999. *Psychopharmacology of Antipsychotics.* London: Martin Dunitz.

Sewell, R. 2012. Latuda: "Procognitive" or Pro-Profit? The Carlat Report Psychiatry.

Stetka, B. 2013. A Guide to DSM-5. *Medscape Multispeciality*, medscape.com

Surman, C.B.H., R. Weisler. 2006. The state of the art treatment for pediatric and adolescent ADHD, medscape.com.

Terr, L. C. 1991. Childhood traumas: an outline and overview. *American Journal of Psychiatry*. 148:10–20.

Thase, M.E., R.H. Howland. 1995. Biological processes in depression: an updated review and integration. In *Handbook of Depression*. E. E. Beckham and W. R. Leber, eds. New York: Guilford Press.

Torrey, E.F. 2001. *Surviving Schizophrenia: A Manual for Families, Consumers, and Providers*. 4th Edition. New York: Quill.

Tucker, G. 2003 Antidepressants still don't seem to make a difference in bipolar depression. *Journal Watch Psychiatry*. 9:2.

Tucker, G. 2003. SSRIs during pregnancy: another view. *Journal Watch Psychiatry*. 9:7.

U.S. Food and Drug Administration. Antidepressant Use in Children, Adolescents, and Adults, fda.gov.

Wegmann, J. 2012. Psychopharmacology: Straight Talk on Mental Health Medications. 2nd Edition. Eau Claire, WI: Premier Publishing & Media

Wehrenberg, M. 2012. The 10 Best-Ever Anxiety Management Techniques Workbook. New York: W.W. Norton & Company.

White, R.F. 2006. Pharmacologic advances in the treatment of ADHD in adults: an expert interview with Richard H. Weisler, MD. Medscape Psychiatry & Mental Health 11(1), medscape.com.

White, R.F. 2006. Quality of life and treatment outcomes with once-daily medications for ADHD: an expert interview with Joseph Biederman, MD. Medscape Psychiatry & Mental Health. 11(1), medscape.com.

Wooten, J., J. Galavis. 2005. Polypharmacy: Keeping the Elderly Safe, rnweb.com.

Zetin, M., and Tate, D. 1999. *The Psychopharmacology Sourcebook*. Lincolnwood, IL: Lowell House.

Resources Websites

Agency for Healthcare Research & Quality, ahrq.gov

American Academy of Child and Adolescent Psychiatry, aacap.org

American Psychiatric Association, psych.org

National Council on Patient Information and Education, talkaboutrx.org National Institute of Mental Health, National Institutes of Health, nimh.nih.gov

National Mental Health Information Center, Substance Abuse and Mental Health Services (SAMHSA), U.S. Department of Health and Human Services, mentalhealth.samhsa.gov

U.S. Food and Drug Administration, fda.gov

World Health Organization, who.int

Index

CE Test Options & Information

Title: Psychopharmacology: Straight Talk on Mental Health Medications, Third Edition

Presented by: JOSEPH F WEGMANN, PHARM.D., LCSW

Product Number: 083825

CE Release Date: 7/1/2015

CE Test Options - Please read each option carefully:

1 - If you've already purchased the Online CE Test, please click on the link below. Log-in to your account and access the CE Test. Upon completion, you'll receive real-time grading & results!

http://www.pesi.com/ceinfo/access/

2 - To purchase and take the Online CE Test, please click on the link below. Save $10 and have real-time grading & results!

http://www.pesi.com/ceinfo/purchase/60135171

3 - To purchase, download, print and complete the (paper version) CE Test, click on the link below. You'll have access to the CE Test in PDF format. Please allow 4-6 weeks for mail, grading & results. A $10 processing fee is included in the price.

http://www.pesi.com/ceinfo/manual/60135171

If you have any questions, please feel free to contact our customer service department at 1.800.844.8260.
**PESI, Inc. offers continuing education programs and products under the brand names PESI, PESI HealthCare, PESI Rehab, Meds-PDN, HealthEd and Ed4Nurses. PESI, Inc., 3839 White Ave, Eau Claire WI, 54703